CARING FOR YOURSELF ~ CARING FOR OTHERS:
THE ULTIMATE BALANCE

First Edition
Third Printing

Diann B. Uustal, R.N., M.S., Ed.D.
President, Educational Resources in HealthCare, Inc.
Consulting Educator
Clinical Ethicist

Published by
SeaSpirit Press

Printed by
Narragansett Graphics
Coventry, R.I.

ISBN: 0-9638759-1-4
Library of Congress Catalog Card Number: 97-90862
Third Printing, July 2002

Published & distributed in the United States by:
SeaSpirit Press a division of
Educational Resources in HealthCare, Inc.
Please note there are two offices:

From September through May each year:	From June to August each year:
2168 South Shore Acres Rd.	PO Box 574
Soddy Daisy, TN 37379	Jamestown, RI 02835-0574
Phone: 423-451-0011	Phone: 401-423-1711
Fax: 423-451-0005	Fax: 401-423-1211

Email: dbuethics@aol.com • Website: www.dbuethics.com

For the two years it took to write this book, this verse has been inspiring and inspiriting for me:

The Lord has given me
the tongue of those who are taught
that I may know how to sustain with a word
those who are weary.
Isaiah 50:4

This book is dedicated with love to the people in my life
who have influenced me the most about caring from the heart
and the joy it brings
Beryl and Charles, my Mom and Dad,
Tom, my husband,
and Kristy and Katie our daughters

and to caregivers from many professions and walks of life
who know the joy and sacrifice of caring and serving.

I hope you find this book refreshing and that it encourages you
to care for yourself as well as you care for others.

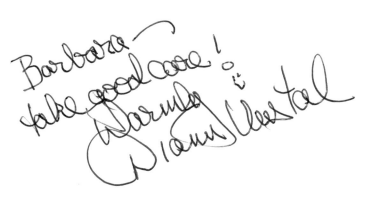

◆ *Acknowledgements* ◆

I am grateful to many people who have shaped my life and my thinking about the importance and necessity of caring for myself so that I can care for others;

to my grandmother and mother for being the best two nurses and nurturers one could grow up modeling;

to my father for his quiet wisdom, wise counsel, and strength of character;

to the happy memory of my father-in-law who was the most compassionate healer-physician I know;

to my husband, Tom, for his constant love, gift of encouragement, and loving reminders and kindness when I'm out of balance;

to our daughters, Kristy and Katie, for allowing me to express and refine the love between a mother and her precious children, no matter what their ages;

to Sid Simon, the most influential professor I've had, who in my eyes and heart will always be the master of teaching people to stay in balance and do what they value;

to John, my lifetime friend, schoolmate, and counsel who sees the best in me when I need it most;

to Jan, whose gift of presence even long distance is inspiring;

and to Jesus Christ without whose personal relationship I would be totally out of balance and whose name is placed at the bottom of this list, not out of forgetfulness, but because of the foundation He offers me.

♦ *Table of Contents* ♦

♦ *Introduction* ♦

Today . . .

Relax.
Taste, touch, hear, see everything
as if for the first time.
Count stars.
Indulge yourself.
Go barefoot.
Take your time.
Let go of a worry.
Take a chance.
Hope.
Play.
Relive a memory.
Dare to dream.
Watch the clouds.
Laugh out loud.
Try. Try again.
Create a joy.
Be kind to yourself.
Be you.

Have you heard the expression, "Today is the first day of the rest of your life?" To what extent does this describe your lifestyle? Are you living each day with a sense of wonder and pleasure or merely going through the motions? How many people do you know that are merely existing and not living?

If there is anything a caregiver can learn from his/her profession of nursing, medicine, social work, or pastoral care, it's that life is precious. There's no guarantee that you'll be on the planet next week or next year. As caregivers we witness and learn from people who are compelled to re-evaluate their lives in the face of a crisis. They tell us time and time again: "Don't sweat the small stuff...and most everything is small stuff." "You learn what's really important when something goes wrong with your health." "Learn to count your blessings and not your burdens."

Why does it seem to take a personal crisis for most of us

to get our priorities straight? What will it take for you to slow down and enjoy life more? How do you want to create today? Today isn't going to happen twice. How do you want it to unfold?

This is a book for caregivers. It's about *caring for yourself* and the *balance* that's involved when you interact with family, friends and are actively involved with your career. It's about meeting your own needs and having enough energy to care for others in your personal as well as professional life. Even more importantly it's about creating a balanced life, not just regaining the balance.

It's about common sense, being gentle on yourself, taking *"time-outs,"* and creating an *inner simplicity*. It's about responsibility for your own well being, and participating in the *"re-creational" therapy* that each of us as busy caregivers needs. It's an invitation to *"be-friend" yourself*, do some *"mental housecleaning"* and to examine *life that often seems to be on fast forward.*

It's full of introspective questions, wellness principles, and strategies that offer simple yet powerful lessons for personal change. Some of the questions appear so simple at first glance, yet become more provocative as you explore your responses, attitudes and values and what they reveal. I hope these introspective strategies serve as a mirror for personal reflection and a springboard for enhancing your self care and overall wellness.

It's written in such a way that even if you only have a few minutes to pick it up, it will encourage you, ask you to think about the balancing act we all experience, and offer strategies that can help you create a more balanced life.

I trust you'll enjoy the book and that it will make you think. I hope it serves as a *wake up call* for some of you, *for others a gentle reminder*, and for some a *confirmation that you're on the right track*. Most importantly, I hope it encourages you to act on what you discover or re-learn. I hope it will be a book that no matter when you pick it up or how many times you've leafed through it's pages, that you'll learn from it again and again.

Take care!

For yourself and for the people in your life.

✦ Caring For Yourself — Caring For Others: The Ultimate Balance ✦

Naturally, each of us wants to be known as a caring person. Intuitively, we value caring as a virtuous characteristic in ourselves and others and a positive quality that ought to be inherent in our relationships, especially those that are most precious. We know that caring is a cornerstone value that shapes the nature and quality of our relationships and a cardinal indicator of healthy relationships. We also understand cognitively and experientially that it takes energy to care for others in a consistent and genuine way.

So whether you are a nurse, a parent in your home, social worker, physician, physician's assistant, pastor, day care provider for adults or children, an exercise physiologist, or volunteer, this book and this question is especially for you:

How do you take care of yourself
in order to be effective in caring for others
and involved in caring relationships?

In addition to being caring individuals, many of us have chosen to be professional caregivers and assume caregiving responsibilities outside of our home, family life, and personal friendships. As professionals we embrace the philosophy that caring is both a traditional and contemporary value and ethic in nursing as well as other caregiving arts and sciences. Yet,

how many of us are as good at caring for ourselves
as we are at meeting the needs of others?

It's time the ethic of caring was expanded to include caring for the caregiver, as well as the more traditional emphasis on the patient's or client's needs. The truth is,

before you can care for others well,
in your personal or professional life,
you must first know how to care for yourself.

I believe we must learn to put first things first and attend to our own body, mind, and spirit before we are able to minister effectively to other people's body, mind, and spirit.

This book is *an invitation to interact with the material and to take some time for yourself and for contemplating what is of value to you.* If you merely read the words you will miss the opportunity to more *carefully examine the balance between caring for yourself and caring for others.*

So read with a pen in hand and complete the exercises that are of interest to you. Write in the spaces provided, the margins, or on a separate piece of paper and spend some time thinking about the questions, exercises, and your responses. As the title of the book implies, caring for yourself and caring for others is the ultimate balance. It's up to you to decide whether a balancing act or a more balanced life is your goal. You are the only one who can change this part of your life.

I hope this book serves as a mirror for personal reflection and a springboard for action that will add to the quality of your life and enhance your relationships! I trust it will give you ideas that will help you put first things first and attend to your own body, mind, and spirit so that you are more able to care for and interact with others.

♦ *The "Fundamentals" Of Nursing* ♦

Caring is the cornerstone of nursing's moral art, science, the profession's code of ethics, and the foundation of each nurse's practice. It is the ethic of care that all nurses and other caregivers share no matter what their clinical specialty, management expertise, teaching commitments, or research responsibilities. It's the cardinal value that connects us together, directs us toward a common goal, and one of the qualities we use to assess a caregiver's moral competency and character.

Caring is rooted in the ethical principle of beneficence, or the obligation to do good, and is expressed in the virtue of benevolence. It is nursing's proud tradition, principal value, contemporary commitment, and vision for healthcare reform and delivery of qualitative patient-focused care. Understandably, caregivers have been taught to focus on and direct this ethic of caring toward the patient or client and family. This is appropriate; however, I believe *the concept of caring needs to be expanded to incorporate a more contemporary vision of caring which includes caring for the caregiver.*

As we quickly approach the twenty-first century and continue to be confronted by the myriad changes taking place in healthcare, it's time we reflect individually and collectively as a profession on the "fundamentals" of nursing. Recall for a moment the fundamentals of nursing textbook you used and the professor who taught the fundamentals course. You secretly might have thought s/he was "over the hill," but the course and text were designed to introduce you to the basic values and obligations you have as a nurse. I'd be willing to bet that there was not even a single chapter, let alone a book, that was devoted to the primary responsibility we have to "take care" in order to care effectively and therapeutically.

The primary thesis for this extended vision of caring and for this entire book is deceptively simple, but by no means simplistic:

> **In order to care effectively**
> **and therapeutically for others,**
> **you must first know how to care for yourself.**

This is true whether you are talking about being a responsive and caring member of your family or you're a professional caregiver. In other words,

> *caring for the caregiver*
> *is an essential and necessary prerequisite*
> *to caring for others.*

I consider these statements to be first steps toward effective caring and expressions of central concepts and core values in personal relationships as well as in the profession of nursing and other caregiving professions. There is a deep and rewarding personal joy and satisfaction in caring for others; however, in order to do this we must learn to put first things first.

Yet how many chapters in our fundamentals of nursing, professional arts, or leadership textbooks are devoted to exploring these ideas? How many offered practical strategies for exploring the *balance between self care and caring for others* and teach us how to care for ourselves in order to therapeutically care for others? Did your professors of nursing discuss and model the balance between self care and caring for others in order to prepare you for the demands of practice? For that matter, were many of us encouraged to explore this important arena as a matter of personal growth and development so that we could lead a more balanced, enriched life? Far too few articles and chapters are published on caring from this broader perspective even though caring as a concept has emerged in the nursing literature with new dimensions and added prestige. Even at the present time there are no texts other than this one that are devoted to discussing the importance of caring for the caregiver or that offer practical strategies that will enhance an individual's ability to examine and accomplish this. Self care is a legitimate and necessary facet of caring for others in a professional environment or in a personal relationship and must be carefully considered and thoughtfully balanced.

♦ *"Common Sense" And "Time-Out" For The Caregiver* ♦

Caring for yourself so you can care for others, staying in balance with self care, and focusing on your needs from a body, mind, and spirit perspective may seem to be a simple enough ideas for enhancing wellness. Perhaps you'd be comfortable calling them "common sense," but you know what's said about common sense. It isn't all that common! You can have a string of degrees at the end of your name, and not one lick of common sense. There's a delicate balance between caring for others too much, maybe even at your own expense, and by not responding to your own needs, and not caring enough because you don't want to get too emotionally involved. The fact is, too few of us as caregivers take time-out to care for ourselves and we seem to have learned relatively few strategies for creating a good balance. If "time-out" can be declared in the midst of a sporting event, we can certainly learn to use it as a strategy in our everyday lives.

Why do you think so many of us continue to pay little attention to caring for ourselves as a first response? Possibly it's the conflicting messages we've heard about "selfishness" and "self-respect," or it's a protective strategy, a gender related issue in our culture, or an unhealthy habit. Perhaps we need to learn to give ourselves permission to put first things first and care for ourselves first so we can respond to others more effectively. A more contemporary message concerning healthy caring is that taking time to care for yourself is evidence of self respect, and it will enable you to care for others out of a full well rather than an empty one. I believe this more balanced attitude toward self care is a necessary prerequisite to caring empathetically for others.

Caring for yourself and declaring time out in order to be able to care for others more effectively is not only common sense; it's also a spiritual principle found as a tenant in numerous faiths. It's found in Scripture in the Judeo-Christian culture, as well as in other religions such as Buddhism and in the Native American tradition. No matter what the spiritual orientation, the principle is expressed in surprisingly similar ways and it encourages you to "love your neighbor as yourself" (Matthew 19:19). When you think about it, you realize that the preposition as is very impor-tant and gives us insight. It means "equal to," "like," or "the same as" we care for ourselves. It does not mean "more than" or "less than." This principle urges us to love and care for our-selves, not only for our own good, but also for other people's benefit. It's a principle that asks that we put ourselves first so that we can have enough energy to care for others and that we care for ourselves at least equally to the way we care for others.

In his book, The Secret of Staying in Love, John Powell said it this way: "...it's a package deal. You have two people you must love: yourself and your neighbor." The way I figure it, if Christ went into the desert to pray and prepare for his daily demands, maybe it would be good judgment for me to put first things first too, in order to be prepared for my work and relation-ships.

It seems many of us care for others far more diligently than we care for ourselves. This is a dynamic and often tentative balance at best and you can often see people at opposite ends of the self care--other care continuum rather than somewhere in the middle. If you care for others and neglect your own needs, this is an imbalance that *over time* can lead to frustration, resentment, and even burnout. On the other hand, if you care for yourself first to the exclusion of others, and *typically* put your own needs and desires ahead of other relationships, this is also an imbalance. Many would label this type of individual or lifestyle narcissistic or hedonistic.

Of course, on any given day anyone could be off balance, but that's temporary and not what we're talking about. The equilibrium we are concentrating on is associated with lifestyle choices and behaviors. It's a focus on creating a balanced life and not just being satisfied with a balancing act, and some people are more willing than others to settle for a balancing act until some event becomes a wake-up call. Nurses and often many women (this does not exclude men) in our culture can easily fall into the pattern of responding to others and neglecting their own needs because of their role as caregivers and gender and cultural expectations and messages. Too many of us run at a fast pace and less frequently take the time for the necessary refreshment we need so that we can continue to be and share all that we are. Sure, you can focus almost exclusively for a while on other's needs; however, one thing is certain: If you do not take time to care for yourself you will find that on a personal, as well as a professional level, you will have less to give and share with your family, patients, friends, and colleagues.

It's no secret that the demands of professional caregiving are stressful and potentially tiring and costly for caregivers no matter what their role or responsibilities or profession. There is increasing evidence that professionals are pressured with myriad ethical issues, value conflicts, rapid changes in contemporary healthcare and in the delivery system. Research indicates many experienced nurses are leaving the profession and there are fewer people choosing nursing as a career. Hospitals report increasing difficulty in both the retention and recruitment of talented, insightful, competent practitioners. Combine this picture with the fact that nurses traditionally have been conditioned to have low self esteem, to neglect their own concerns in favor of meeting the needs of others, and are less highly regarded in the system as healers and professionals than other caregivers. Because of these changes and pressures, there has never been a more important time to emphasize that self care is vital to caring for others.

Many of us will nod in agreement
that caring for the caregiver is important,
but will we make the changes required
for an effective balance
between meeting our own needs
and other's needs?

Some people will still interpret caring for one's self as selfishness; others will acknowledge self care as a necessity and an attitude of self respect. Some folks will even read about tools that can help them make healthy changes, but will fail to incorporate them into their lifestyles. Unfortunately, the importance of caring for oneself is a deceptively simple notion, often elusive, and seems less apparently imperative the more demanding our personal and professional lives become.

Regretfully, most professionals were not exposed to the common sense and basic concepts about self care, and it was rarely taught or discussed in any of our caregiver curricula. We prepared men and women for the demands and discipline of professions that specialize in the art and science of human caring and healing from a holistic perspective and then neglect to teach them to care for themselves, too. As a nurse you need to be clear that you are a significant part of the caring, healing process, and relationship; however, you're less effective with patients, clients, and their families if you're in need of "intensive care" yourself.

I believe nursing can be even more effective as an art and science if nurses take time out to care for the caregiver. Healthy caring is a reflection of a qualitative balance between meeting your own needs and the needs of others. Any asset such as caring can become a liability. It's a matter of proportion and each of us must individually work out the right balance regarding this value and vision of healthy caring. This book is rich with ideas and strategies.

Most of us would readily agree that "an ounce of prevention is worth a pound of cure," and "a stitch in time saves nine." They're two familiar expressions with a ring of truth that many of us would do well to recall. Taking time to care for yourself before you are burned out, rusted out, or resentful, over-extended, and out of energy is essential. Many of us are in need of intensive care, but wait until we are in critical condition to attend to our own body, mind, and spirit.

What are some simple things you need to do to restore a sense of balance in your personal as well as your professional life? Read on and you'll find some practical ideas and strategies to help you lead a more balanced life and not just maintain a balancing act!

Don't relegate self care to a distant second place.
Caring for the caregiver is not an option, it's a necessity!
Take Care!

◆ *A Balancing Act Or A Balanced Life?* ◆

A balancing act or a balanced life. Which phrase more accurately describes your style and your approach to life? Balance can be an elusive concept and experience for some of us. Does it lead you to picture yourself as a person walking on a tightrope? As you watch yourself, are you walking with or without a net? Do you just sometimes or very often feel that way in your personal life? What about your professional life?

<u>**Webster's Dictionary**</u> **defines "balance" as:**

Balance.   (bal.ance) n.
1.   an instrument for weighing; typically a bar poised or swaying on a central support.
2.   a state of bodily equilibrium.
3.   a stable mental or psychological state; emotional stability.
4.   a harmonious or satisfying arrangement or proportion of parts or elements, as in a design.

Balance is one of the key concepts in this book and is essential to wellness and self care. What does it mean for you to be in balance? Think about it and write your response here:

 Here are some questions that will get you thinking more about balance in your life and will help clarify what's important to you. Jot your initial responses in the spaces provided and use them as food for thought. When you come back to them again, get really involved and use them as journal entries and write more lengthy responses.

- Do you consider your life to be balanced?

- Which phrase, a "balancing act" or a "balanced life" more accurately describes your lifestyle?

- Which would you prefer?

- What's difficult for you to balance? Be as specific as you can.

- What's harder for you to keep in balance, your personal or professional life?

- What are the reason(s) for the imbalance(s)?

- What can you do or what attempts have you made to bring yourself back into balance?

- How successful have you been?

- What do you need to continue to do in order to change the imbalance(s)?

- What do you need to learn or re-learn in order to bring more balance into your life?

- What are you doing well?

- What did you have to do to get yourself there? What agreements do you have to establish with yourself in order to create a more balanced lifestyle?

♦ Caring for Yourself and Others: A Delicate Balance ♦

In your personal, family and professional life, you must realistically balance meeting your needs with meeting the needs of others. This is especially important for a caregiver since meeting other's needs understandably has priority in certain circumstances or relationships. What we're focusing on here are your patterns, not specific roles.

In order to care for the people in your personal life effectively over time you must first know how to care for yourself. Respond to the following questions as you reflect on your patterns of self care:

 Think about your personal, family, and career commitments and the way you spend your time, energy, and the way you feel as you answer the following question: **Do you think your life is balanced?**

On a scale of 1-10, put an X on the line to indicate how conscientious you are in caring for others.

1_____**10**

Meeting the needs of others

On a scale of 1-10, put an X on the line to indicate how conscientious you are in caring for yourself.

1_____**10**

Meeting my own needs

What are some **things that throw you off balance**?

1.

2.

3.

4.

5.

List some things you usually do to **try to keep your balance**:

1.

2.

3.

4.

5.

Identify some things you could do <u>more of</u> to stay in balance:

On a daily basis: This week:
1.   1.
2.   2.
3.   3

This month: This year:
1.   1.
2.   2.
3.   3.

What are some things you could do <u>less of</u> which would help you keep your balance:

On a daily basis: This week:
1.   1.
2.   2.
3.   3.

This month: This year:
1.   1.
2.   2.
3.   3.

What are some strategies you've been successful using that have helped you stay in balance?

1.

2.

3.

4.

5.

Look at your strategies for staying in balance. If you're in need of some rest and relaxation now, be sure to pick a strategy that will refresh you immediately and not one that's more appropriate for a longer block of time that's available in the future.

Here are some things other caregivers say about **what throws them off balance**: Do any sound familiar?

- "There's never enough time to do everything I 'should' do, never mind what I want to do."

- "Unexpected situations or demands."

- "Escalating job requirements in an unresponsive and overly demanding work environment."

- "Writing lists constantly and then trying to accomplish too much in too little time. Then I beat myself up for not getting everything done I said I would."

- "I have young grandchildren and my kids need my help, but I have no life of my own."

Here are some ideas caregivers have shared about **how they try to stay in balance**:

- "I have a friend who 'schedules' her pleasurable times and sticks to it. I need to plan ahead for fun with my schedule and life, but I never do. I let everything else takes precedence. I'm going to change this."

- "I write long letters to one of my lifetime friends. She's a confidant and she does the same with me. We save the letters. It's like a record of our development and has helped both of us tremendously."

- "I work on our family photo album when I want to recall the good times."

- "I live in a cold environment and I'm always planning for my spring vegetable garden. I'm saving for a greenhouse addition to our house so I can grow things in the colder months too."

- "I watch M*A*S*H* re-runs on video and laugh out loud!"

- "Sorting through my favorite cookbooks and planning to try new recipes cures my mood immediately and it's great when we enjoy my creative adventures together."

 "Self love, my liege, is not so vile a sin as self neglect."
—Shakespeare's <u>King Henry V</u>

♦ "Put Your Own Oxygen Mask On First!" ♦

When you travel on airplanes an announcement you hear before every departure bears a noteworthy message and has merit for caregivers:

"...In case of an emergency during the flight, please put your own oxygen mask on first, and then assist others who may need it."

To a caregiver, this message may sound incongruous. Haven't we learned the lesson of caring for and being responsible for others first so well that we often ignore our own needs? Maybe there's another lesson worth learning. To some of us it will sound radical, to others more familiar.

The message is simple but not simplistic: healthy caring is a balancing act. It's a balance between meeting your own needs and the needs of others. In order to care for others you must first be able to care for yourself. You will then have more energy to care for others. Here are some introspective questions that are important for you to carefully consider.

- How do you **feel** when you read or hear that "In order to care for others you must first know how to care for your self?"

- What are the first **thoughts** you have or what do you **say** to yourself?

- What are the messages you've heard and learned about putting yourself first?

- What do you need to do more conscientiously to **take care** and "**put your own oxygen mask on first?**"

In the space provided, list the things you **typically do to stay in balance** between meeting your own needs and the needs of others.

1.

2.

3.

4.

5.

6.

7.

Fill in the following statement as many times as you can. Don't edit your thinking, just jot your ideas down.

In order to stay healthy and able to care for others, I need to. . .

1.

2.

3.

4.

5.

6.

7.

8.

9.

10.

Something to think about:
*Does putting yourself first feel
like selfishness or self-respect?*

*"Treasure and care for yourself. Then
your love and care for others will flow
out of a full well without the limitations
of your own needs."*
—*Diann Uustal*

◆ *Things I Love to Do* ◆

"Quality of life" is a term many of us in health care are familiar with. But right now we're not talking about a patient's quality of life, we're talking about yours. Quality of life is a subjective evaluation and it's enhanced when you do the things you love to do. What makes you happy and brings joy to your life? What do you really enjoy doing?

This exercise gives you the chance to identify some of these things. In the space below, list as many of the things you love to do as you can think of. Don't edit your responses.

"Code"	Things I Love to Do
_____	1.
_____	2.
_____	3.
_____	4.
_____	5.
_____	6.
_____	7.
_____	8.
_____	9.
_____	10.

✳️ Now that you've written your list of what you do love to do, let's see what you can learn when you analyze the list. I call the "coding" our list. Place the appropriate letter(s) next to the things on your list which indicate the following. You can have more than one letter next to any of the items on your list:

P	primarily a <u>physical</u> activity
E	typically <u>emotionally</u> refreshing
S	usually <u>social</u>
Sp	<u>spiritually</u> uplifting
I	essentially an <u>intellectual</u> pursuit you enjoy
MO	you meed to do <u>more often</u>
A	for the things you typically do <u>alone</u>
O	you do this with <u>others</u>
B	you'd like to be <u>better</u> at
R	<u>relaxing</u> for you
CR	involves elements of <u>calculated risk</u>
U	this activity is <u>unconventional</u>
V	you've been <u>validated</u> or praised for
C	you do this <u>consistently</u>
SR	adds to your <u>self renewal</u> and "re-creation"
HH	you love to do this but it's a <u>health hazard</u>
L	makes you <u>laugh</u> out loud and lighten up
SE	<u>sheer enjoyment</u> is why you do this
EN	gets you <u>energized</u> and recharged
M	enhances your <u>mood</u>, enthusiasm
$	for anything on your list that costs less than a compact disc
75	you'll still be able to do this when you're 75
F	it's <u>frivolous</u> and fun

☐ **Prioritize your four favorite activities. These are the activities that if you had to give them up your quality of life would be influenced.**

☐ **Date each of your top four activities (approximately) to indicate when you last did this activity.**

☐ **Next to your favorite four activities, identify a couple of benefits, pleasures, or satisfactions you gain from doing them.**

☐ **Write the name of the person(s) you'd most like to do this activity with next to these activities.**

✳ Now look at your list again and how you coded it and think about the following ideas to get you started on discovering what you've learned or re-learned about how you care for yourself.

Did you notice that the first five ways of examining and coding your list were based on what we've learned from holistic health? Holistic health encourages us to take responsibility for our own health and to remember that there are *physical, emotional, intellectual, social and spiritual aspects* of ourselves. Ignoring your needs in any of these vital areas is could cause you to be out of balance in caring for yourself. This concept of whole-person caring is not unfamiliar to caregivers. We encourage each other to care for patients in this way. Too often, what is foreign to many of us, is that we attend to our own needs from a holistic perspective much less effectively than we meet our client's needs.

For example, many of us know that we should be doing certain things physically for our health such as exercising at least three times a week at eighty percent of our target heart rate based on our age as recommended by the American Heart Association. Yet how many of us who believe this health tip actually value it enough to consistently incorporate it into our behavior? My professor and mentor, Sid Simon, taught "Do what you value. Value what you do." For how many of us is this an accurate description of our wellness behavior? The significant difference between what we believe and what we value is *action*. Many of us give lip service to the importance of taking care of ourselves. Fewer of us take consistent action.

What is the result of inconsistent self care while you continue to meet the needs of others in your personal and professional life? I believe this could lead to burn out whether you're a lay person or a caregiving professional. You appropriately focus on other's needs, but you cannot consistently continue to meet other's needs unless you are able to satisfy your own. It is out of this refreshment and balance, that you are able to give to and care for others! Caring for yourself and others is a delicate balance and each person's balance is personal and unique.

As you continue to examine your list, what did you discover in regard to the emotional (E) things on your list? Are you doing too little in terms of caring for yourself spiritually (SP)? Do you need more alone (A) time to refresh? Are you cultivating enough activities and interests you can continue doing in the future (F) when you're fifteen to twenty years older?

 As you look over your list and how you've categorized it, what can you discover about your patterns of self care? What do you need to be doing more/less of to enhance your wellness? What do you need to do less/more of to bring yourself into balance? As you reflect on this information, see the self contract in this book.

 You know how you make myriad lists of things to do and then try to accomplish them? Why not make a list of things you love to do and hold yourself to accomplishing these things on your list in order to enhance your quality of life?

The value in an exercise like this is in careful reflection on what you've learned.

 Complete the following sentences and see what else you can discover about your patterns of self care.

I learned that I _____

I realize I need to _____

I'm aware that. _____

I re-affirmed that I _____

I discovered _____

I am pleased that I _____

I found out _____

I appreciated that I _____

Something that surprised me was _____

Your own statement: _____

When you plan your time, put private time, family time and leisure time first. Then schedule everything else around these.

William James, a noted psychologist who wrote about change, advised people who wanted to make changes in their lives to:

"Start immediately, tell everyone what you're doing so they'll support and encourage you, and make no exceptions."

Simple criteria, but by no means simplistic. Go ahead, try it!

Enjoy Life.
This isn't a dress rehearsal.

♦ *Quality of Life* ♦

Quality of life is an expression we hear in health care that usually refers to someone else's life. But what about our own? What are the things you can do to create wellness and more quality in your life and in other's lives?

This exercise is a compilation of practical ideas that can help you create more balance in your life.

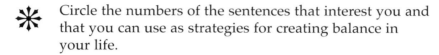 Circle the numbers of the sentences that interest you and that you can use as strategies for creating balance in your life.

1. Lighten up! Do a few things backwards and upside-down to change your "routine" and wake up the robot in you.
2. When you're feeling overwhelmed, do some "strength training." Identify your strengths and assets.
3. Sincerely compliment or praise your spouse, child, friend, or colleague. Praise them publicly. Now do the same for someone you don't particularly care for.
4. Choose a fitness program that works for you. Working out is not punishment for a body that's not a "10," it's a sign of self care. Your body is a temple. Treat it with respect.
5. Speak gently to your inner self. You need encouragement, appreciation, and healthy self talk.
6. Send yourself to your room. Learn to retreat for relaxation and re-creation.
7. Catch others or yourself doing something well and right and validate yourself or the other person.
8. Refuse to listen to negative messages—your own and others. Change the channel or play a new tape.
9. Think of some creative ways to reach out the people in your life and think of some ways you could ask them to touch yours.
10. Play at least one noncompetitive game where everyone wins.
11. Exercise your spirit.
12. Start something brand new—today.
13. Make plans to see someone you've been missing. Rekindle a relationship.
14. Admire yourself and celebrate the gifts you've been given.
15. Spread good news.

16. Do something unnecessarily nice for someone....and for yourself.
17. Breathe deeply and take a few minutes to be aware of what you're grateful for. Cultivate an attitude of gratitude.
18. Dream of what you want to be when you grow up.
19. Expect miracles. Create miracles.
20. Eat something inspiring.
21. Be good to yourself. You can't be there for someone else unless you take care of yourself. Learn to love yourself "as" (which means equal to) your neighbor.
22. Take time and space for yourself so that you're not burned out or burned up when others need something from you.
23. Pay attention to and experience your feelings. Then decide what you want to do with them: just feel them, express them, or act on them.
24. Stop harassing yourself. You do this when you need or want something to change. Figure out what you're really saying to yourself.
25. When you can't think straight....stop thinking....and start paying attention to your feelings.
26. When you're feeling stressed, slow down your thinking movements, and speech.
27. If crying helps, cry. If it's not good timing, promise yourself the time to cry later. Be sure to keep your promise.
28. Be your own inspiration.
29. Recall a precious moment. Let go of a painful one.
30. Take time to enjoy the benefit of completing a project...and a job well done.
31. Do something playful. You're never too old to play!
32. Treat yourself like your own best friend.
33. When the going gets tough—rest, but don't quit!
34. Learn to accept yourself as you are. Regard others in the same way.
35. Don't compare yourself to another person. Compare yourself to your own potential.
36. When things are rough, tell someone and let them care for you. Two are always better than one.
37. Search for and cultivate inner peace. It's a blessing to you and those around you.
38. Recall and celebrate precious moments.
39. Be solution oriented rather than problem oriented. Be a part of the solution and not a part of the problem.

40. Think of a special friend who loves you for who you are—and pass along the gift of positive regard.
41. Pat your pet and get some "pet therapy." Pets help you pay attention to right now.
42. Get involved in some volunteer work in some area other than your caregiving profession.
43. Pay attention and learn to respond to your intuitive self.
44. When your heart speaks, listen carefully and take good notes.
45. Be pro-active not re-active in relation to issues that confront you.
46. Forgive someone not so much for their sake, but for your own.
47. Happiness is a choice. Practice happiness.
48. Don't forget, no one died and left you in charge of the universe.
49. Stay in the room. Try to live in the present and not in the past or the future.
50. Don't "push a river." Allow things to unfold the way they should.
51. Tomorrow is promised to no one. Live today qualitatively.
52. Enjoy the company of healthy friends. Avoid the people who drag you down especially when you're low on energy.
53. Think about the things, people places that bring happiness to your life.
54. Create joy in your life more often and when things get tough, recall what brings you joy and relish it. Gain strength and energy from it and go on.
55. Set aside a space of time where you have no schedule and nothing that has to be done except what you want to do, even if it's just for a short time.
56. Learn to say to yourself "Every need is not my calling or responsibility."
57. Schedule therapeutic massages to help you relax and decrease stress as a regular part of your self care and wellness. Don't save it for vacations only.
58. Try not to over-react to a difficult situation and let the situation get the best of you.
59. Select a particular cuisine. Then cook, experiment, and dine accordingly with some other adventurous folks.

 "Whatever is true, noble, right, pure, lovely, admirable—if anything is excellent or praiseworthy—think about these things."
—Phil 4:8

◆ R X : T a k e C a r e ! ◆

Too often, for caregivers, caring for oneself is a low priority. Meeting the needs of family, friends, patients and colleagues as well as keeping up with myriad obligations command our attention, time and energy.

If you don't take the time to take care every once in a while, there's probably no harm done. However, if neglecting self care is a more predominant pattern, the results can be detrimental. You may find yourself chronically tired, feeling there's no time for yourself, burned out, or worse—angry and disillusioned.

Some of us say, "I have no time to care for myself!" That should be a signal for reflection. Here are three things to think about:

- **We all have 24 hours a day: no more no less.**

- **How you prioritize your time is based on what you value or feel is important. Is caring for yourself important?**

- **If you don't take care of yourself, who's "supposed" to?**

Why is it that some of us think taking care of oneself is someone else's responsibility? And when they don't take care of us, why is it that we get angry at them?

In some relationships, taking care of each other is more of a mutual expectation or responsibility; however, people can't read our minds and many of us don't ask for what we need or want. When others don't meet our unexpressed needs or wants, we believe they aren't sensitive or don't really care for us. We might start to feel unappreciated, tell ourselves we must not deserve it, or we're not worth it. These can be sickening messages which erode our own health as well as the quality of our relationships.

So what are you doing to take care of yourself—to "restock your pantry," "refuel," or "reinvest" in yourself in order to revitalize?

In the space provided, **write down the things you typically do to take care.**

1.   2.

3.   4.

5.   6.

7.   8.

9.   10.

Here are some questions for you to think about and respond to:

1. What do you need to do **more of** to take care of yourself? Be as specific as you can.

2. What do you need to do **less of** in order to take care of yourself?

3. Think about a person you know who takes good care of her/himself. What are some of the things this person does to "take care"? Write them down.

4. Ask this person what things s/he does to take care. You may learn some new strategies. Consider this person a "personal trainer"or wellness mentor. Write down the additional ideas they've shared.

5. Ask your mentor to tell you what s/he thinks you could do that would be helpful. Write their suggestions here.

6. Considering what you've identified you could do, and the ideas you've gotten from your personal trainer, what ideas seem as if they would work for you? List them in order of importance.

    •

    •

    •

    •

    •

    •

Keep these in mind and respond to the following questions.

- What's **one thing** you could do to take better care of your-self **today**?

- What's **one thing** you could do to take better care of your-self **this week**?

- What's **one thing** you could do to take better care of your-self **this month**?

- What's **one thing** you could do to take better care of your-self **this year**?

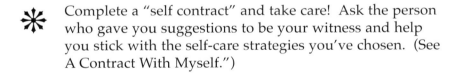 Complete a "self contract" and take care! Ask the person who gave you suggestions to be your witness and help you stick with the self-care strategies you've chosen. (See A Contract With Myself.")

See the exercise "Asking for What You Need and Want." It's a good complement to this exercise.

◆ *" R e a s o n s "   O r   " E x c u s e s " ?* ◆

*People justify not taking care
of themselves for lots of reasons.
Or are they excuses?*

There are differences between reasons and excuses. <u>Webster's</u> states that **reasons** are: "the basis or motive for an action, decision, or conviction; a declaration made to explain them; an underlying fact that provides logical sense; good judgment, sound sense."

Excuses are used to "explain a fault or an offense in hopes of being understood, forgiven, or being able to make allowance for; overlook to serve as justification for, to free as from an obligation or duty."

Ever heard some of these "reasons"? Ever used them yourself?

> **"I have very little free time for myself because I have kids who need shuttling around all the time."**
>
> **"I'm too busy to exercise."**
>
> **"Most of the time I'm too tired after work."**

What are the <u>reasons</u> you don't take care of yourself as well as you could?

1.

2.

3.

4.

5.

Look at the definitions of reasons and excuses once more. Now look at your list of reasons.

- How many of them are really excuses?
- Circle the numbers of the "reasons" that are really "excuses."

Remember, they're excuses if you're using them so that you or others can understand, make allowances for, overlook, or not pay attention to your obligations to yourself.

 To help you continue to clarify the differences between reasons and excuses and think about caring for yourself, answer the following questions:

- Is continuing to refuse to take responsibility for your self care logical?

- Is it good judgment or sound sense?

- How can you justify not taking care of yourself given what you know?

- Where does this pattern come from?

- What messages do you recall learning? Write some of them here.

- What do you get from such a pattern? How does it benefit you?

- What's the price you'll pay for continuing to behave like this?

- Do you believe you'll pay a price, eventually or later?

  Remember: your reasons are excuses if you're using them so that you or others can understand, make allowances for, overlook, or not pay attention to your obligations to yourself.

♦ The "Politics" Of Self Esteem ♦

Self esteem can be simply described as all the beliefs and attitudes you have about yourself. Two things influence your self esteem in a fundamental way:

What you say to yourself and what others say to you.

In addition, your self esteem is shaped by your relationships, the things you do, what you value, your successes, and your failures.

Your mind is never quiet and your internal dialogue or "self talk" is constant. Listen to what you say to and about yourself. Are you positive and encouraging or do you tend to be critical and demanding? What you say to yourself shapes your self esteem tremendously.

In other words, you are what you think and how you think about yourself influences your self concept, behavior, willingness to and interest in caring for yourself, and in turn your ability to care for others. Psychologists report that people behave in ways that are consistent with their self esteem. How you perceive yourself determines what you think you are able to do and what you will try to accomplish.

We all know that if an athlete thinks positively about her/himself before an event it influences performance. The same concept is true for and influences each of us. When you think positively about yourself, your self esteem is strengthened and this has a direct and positive impact on your ability to continue to care for others. You can't minister to people out of an empty well. So how do you replenish your well when it starts running dry?

 You can influence your self esteem and therefore your ability to care by reflecting on questions that focus on positive things about yourself. Here are just a few to get you started. Write your responses in the spaces provided and watch how your ideas change when you reflect on the questions again.

- What are you are good at or best at?

- What do you think people admire most about you?

- Describe yourself. Use whatever adjectives come to mind.

- Now describe yourself again as your best friend would.

- What's the personal achievement or accomplishment you're most proud of?

- What's your most noteworthy professional achievement?

- What makes you special or unique?

- What's the best compliment anyone could give you?

- What would you most like to have your colleagues or friends say about you?

- When you give ourself a "pep talk" what do you say to yourself?

I know, as you respond you feel as if you're bragging! And there are lots of negative messages about people who talk positively about themselves. Sometimes they're called "stuck-up," "arrogant," "conceited," "snotty," "rude," and "pompous." People say "Who does s/he think s/he is?" However, talking positively to and about yourself is not bragging. It is a way of being kind to or gentle on yourself and treating your self sensitively. It will even make you feel good about yourself—what's wrong with feeling good about yourself? It can even positively influence the way you care for others.

Many of us are actually more comfortable with put downs than with praise—from ourselves or others! No wonder it's more typical and we get accustomed to it. But why put yourself down, unfortunately, there are always others who will do it for you! Speak positively to yourself and about yourself!

 "I discovered I am as beautiful as I allow myself to be."
—Deborah Elder Brown
Twentieth Century American Writer

◆ *A f f i r m a t i o n s   A n d   H e a l t h y   S e l f   T a l k* ◆

Are you cultivating a mental garden that has more weeds than flowers?

Affirmations are validating, positive things you say to yourself. They're descriptions of a condition you want to achieve. Affirming yourself is healthy self talk. It's like planting a seed and cultivating it. Think of affirmations as the flowers from your garden that you pick for yourself.

So when you check out your "mental garden," does it have more weeds than flowers? If you had a real garden, you wouldn't intentionally plant weeds in it would you, so why would you sow negative thoughts? Weeds are the put downs or negative self talk. Weeds take away from the beauty of a real garden just like negative self talk erodes your self esteem and confidence.

Since your "internal voice" is never quiet, you should pay attention to what you say to yourself. Is it a critical voice or one that encourages you? Do the messages affirm or put you down? Are they flowers or weeds in your mental garden?

Recognize your negative self talk and the disapproving things you keep telling yourself and work on changing this pattern. Sure you have room for improvement, and you know in what areas better than anyone else, but you will have less energy and desire to change if you're constantly dumping on yourself!

Learn to affirm yourself, you'll really appreciate it! It will enhance your confidence, self esteem, and willingness to take the necessary steps to ensure the changes you want to achieve. Compliment, praise, and validate yourself for who you are and what you do. Speak to yourself positively the way you encourage someone you love. Uplift and encourage yourself with what you say to yourself.

Here are some examples of affirming statements and ideas that will help you get started.

"**I** look and I feel best at 135 pounds." or "I look and feel best when I exercise at least three or four times a week." These are very different messages from, "I'm fat!" or "I can't believe I'm this heavy!" **Affirming statements that concentrate on the desired outcome you want to achieve give you direction.**

You could also take a thought or a quote and turn it into an affirmation. For example, "No one can make you feel inferior without your consent." (Eleanor Roosevelt) Maybe this is one of your favorites and you really believe it, but you catch yourself saying, "He makes me so mad! She makes my blood boil!" Realize that you choose to respond to that situation in that particular way and no one can change that but you. There are many emotions, so try to consciously choose the way in which you would like to respond. Repeat to yourself silently, or out loud, the positive message and maybe the next time your reactions will be more of what you choose. "No one can make me feel anything unless I choose to feel that way." or "I will not allow anyone to make me feel any emotion unless I choose to respond that way." These are more positive message that are healthier for you.

Here's an example of an affirming statement from <u>Dear Stranger,</u> by Catherine Caldwell. "I am developing an interesting, happy human being; the only one I have total control over and the one I've abused and neglected the most." Maybe you'll want to "edit" this for your own use.

My favorite affirmation of all time was penned by my friend and mentor, Sid Simon. It is actually the title of a book he wrote. "I am lovable and capable." You may want to repeat it out loud a few times if you know you're facing a demanding person or situation!

"**I** have all the ability, discipline, energy, resources, and support necessary to accomplish this goal. I will not allow anyone to cause me to doubt my ability, my self, or this aspiration." **This is another example of an affirmation that could be used if**

you're facing a challenge of some kind.

Here's an affirmation a woman in one of my workshops shared. She was recovering from a painful divorce and "practiced" saying this statement out loud: "I have great worth separate from my performance and this is a gift to me as a Christian. I am deeply loved, fully pleasing, accepted and acceptable, and complete in God's eyes." She said when she's really hurting and full of doubts about herself, she takes the card out of her pocket and reads it to herself a few times.

"Today and every day I begin my life anew. I keep my body, mind and soul in balance. My spirit keeps me young. I enjoy and learn from my life." Another workshop participant shared that she read this sentence in an advertisement in a magazine and decided it was a great affirmation!

From these examples you can see that healthy self talk and affirmations are messages that are positive, direct, and speak volumes to you. Be sure to work on phrasing your comments in as positive a way as you can. For example, "I can complete this paper with ease," is even more effective than "This paper will not be hard for me."

Learn and grow from the affirmations and healthy self talk! Then pass along the gift by encouraging and affirming to others.

 Write a couple of affirmations on a 3x5 card and put it in a strategic place where you'll be able to read it several times a day.

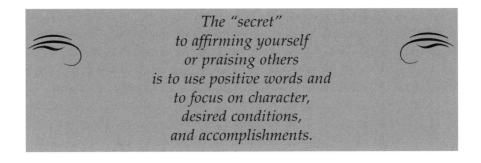

The "secret"
to affirming yourself
or praising others
is to use positive words and
to focus on character,
desired conditions,
and accomplishments.

✦ *I Love Myself The Way I Am* ✦

The following song was written by Jai Joseph & performed by Alliance. It was first shared with me and sung at a Caring for the Caregiver workshop by Shirley Bodie, RN.

I love myself the way I am
There's nothing I need to change
I'll always be the perfect me
There's nothing to rearrange
I'm beautiful & capable
Of being the best me I can
And I love myself just the way I am. . .

I love you just the way you are
There's nothing you need to do
When I feel the love inside myself
It's easy to love you
Behind your fears, your raging tears
I see your shining star
And I love you just the way you are. . .

I love the world the way it is
Cause I can clearly see
That all the things I judge are done
By people just like me
So tell the birth of peace on earth
That only love can bring
And I'll help it grow
By loving everything. . .

I love myself that way I am
And still I want to grow
The change outside can only come
When deep inside I know
I'm beautiful & capable
Of being the best me I can
And I love myself just the way I am
I love my self just the way I am !

- As you read the words of the first stanza of this song, what did you think?

- Do you love yourself the way you are with no changes or are you more typically in the business of "editing" yourself and more critical of yourself?

- What are the things you truly love about yourself?

- What are the things you want to change?

- Do you find that you can think of what you don't like about yourself easier than what you do like?

- Why do you think this happens?

- Where do you think you learned this pattern?

- What will you have to do to change this pattern?

- When you read and reflect on the second verse, do you find that you are more judgmental than you need to be and less unconditional and accepting of other people and their behavior?

- Did you know that what we do not like in ourselves is what we tend to criticize in others? Think of some examples that might reveal this pattern.

- Do you see yourself as "beautiful and capable" like the song says?

- How could we teach this wellness attitude to our children, our friends, ourselves?

As a special project in a graduate course in ethics I taught, three nurses made a commitment to work with fourth grade students in an inner city school as a part of their community outreach requirement. They brought guitars into the classroom and taught the children to sing this song and participate in some values clarifying and self esteem exercises. Their goals were to enhance self esteem, promote an attitude of acceptance of the cultural diversity and uniqueness of each individual, increase caring behaviors and decrease aggressive responses among the children, and improve the tolerance of the differences among the children. It seemed more important than teaching the capitals of the states. I think it is an outstanding example of contemporary nurses enhancing wellness and health promotion in the community!

♦ *Positive Self Talk* ♦

 Talk nicely to yourself!
You'll really appreciate it!

A little positive self talk never hurt anyone. In fact it could help. It could even enhance your self esteem, performance, attitude, energy, or just plain make you feel better about yourself!

❋ Jot down some things you could say to yourself that are affirming, encouraging or validating.

1.

2.

3.

4.

5.

6.

7.

8.

In the space below write down some of the things you say that are critical or negative about yourself.

1.

2.

3.

4.

5.

6.

7.

8.

Was it easier for you to think of the positive or negative things about yourself?

 Psychologists say your mind is never quiet. But self talk can be either affirming or discouraging. Many of us are unnecessarily hard on ourselves or overly critical, so pay attention to what you typically say to yourself.

♦ *Qualities I Like Best About Myself* ♦

Here's a wonderful, simple strategy you can use to examine and enhance your self esteem and influence your ability to care for others more effectively.

Think about the qualities you like best about yourself and use the space provided to record your responses. Perhaps it's easier to get in touch with what you don't like, but that doesn't build self esteem, it erodes it. Concentrate on what lifts your spirits and what you appreciate about yourself. Don't stop writing until you run out of things you like.

"Code"	Qualities I Like Best About Myself:
_____	1.
_____	2.
_____	3.
_____	4.
_____	5.
_____	6.
_____	7.
_____	8.
_____	9.

You can "code" or examine your list more carefully and learn more from what you have identified. Code your list by using the letters or symbols suggested and writing them on the line in front of the numbers on your list:

P   for any physical qualities
E   for emotional qualities
I   for intellectual qualities
S   for social qualities
Sp   for spiritual qualities
W   for qualities you work to maintain
*   to indicate that someone with whom you work or live has recently told you that it is a quality they like about you.
Write two additional qualities you would like to have as characteristics describing yourself
Number the top 3 qualities you want to be known or remembered for the most.
Use a letter or symbol and make up your own way to code your list.

 Here are some additional ideas to help you get more from this exercise:

•   The first five ways of coding your list help you look at yourself from a "whole person" perspective. It makes sense and is essential to care for yourself in each of these areas before you attempt to meet other's needs holistically.

•   What else can you learn from this exercise? Maybe you noticed there are relatively few physical qualities on your list that you really like best about yourself and that this is an area where you are very critical of yourself. This isn't an uncommon issue. Women are particularly critical of themselves from a physical perspective. Maybe you need to focus more on stopping your negative self talk about your physical self and concentrate on what you do appreciate and like.

•   Lastly, look carefully at your list and how you've "coded" it one more time. Complete the following unfinished sentences as you reflect on what you've written.

I found out that I:

I can appreciate that I:

I learned that I:

I discovered that I:

I'm pleased that I:

You already know that you're not always going to feel good about all aspects of yourself. We all have days when we're down on ourselves for different reasons. Sometimes an attitude of critical self evaluation is incentive for self improvement, but a steady attitude of self put downs can erode anyone's self esteem.

So consciously cultivate a positive attitude about yourself. Intentionally recall the things you like best about yourself, your skills and talents. Remember this affects not only your attitudes about yourself, but also your personal relationships with others and your professional caregiving.

Hugh Prather's quote from his journal, <u>Notes to Myself</u> is insightful:

 "The more you know about yourself, and the more positive your self image, the better chance you have of increasing your self esteem and of enjoying a meaningful, happy life."

◆ *Enhancing Your Personal Wellness And Self Esteem* ◆

Here's an exercise with some ideas that could help you construct a wellness care plan and enhance your self esteem. Circle the numbers of the sentences that are important to you. Circle as many as you'd like. Once you have chosen the ideas that are appealing to you, continue reading to discover how each of them can be expanded into a wellness strategy that's practical and effective.

1. Remind yourself and validate yourself for your positive qualities.

2. Be aware of what you do well and what you have done well in the past.

3. Maximize your assets and minimize your liabilities.

4. Identify your strengths and resources and find ways to use them when in new and difficult situations.

5. Don't put yourself down. When you're feeling down, focus on the positive aspects of yourself, rather than negative judgements.

6. Assess difficult situations and concentrate on what you can do differently rather than putting yourself down.

7. Set realistic goals and reward yourself for the progress you make, no matter how small.

8. People can't read your mind! Learn to ask for what you need and want. It will increase the chances you'll receive it!

9. Think and say positive things to yourself...stop negative thoughts that are recurring messages.

10. Be gentle on yourself.

11. Give the gift of encouragement, support, and praise to family and peers...and learn to receive it yourself.

12. Take time for quiet time...find a quiet spot and use it daily for prayer, meditation and re-newing.

13. Take time for "laugh therapy" and time for fun. Schedule it in advance of you have to.

14. Say no. Withdrawing and anger are far more harmful than admitting an inability to do more.

15. Form or join a support group.

16. Examine your complaining...is it complaining that relieves stress or complaining that reinforces stress?

17. Go creative...try a new approach to resolving a problem. Be your own consultant.

18. Learn to take mental health breaks and mini-vacations.

19. Focus on anything but work during your breaks and lunches.

20. Mentally inventory all the good things that have happened during the day and the things you are thankful for.

21. Learn to say "I choose" rather than "I should" and "I won't" rather than "I can't."

22. Clarify the difference between self-respect (taking time for yourself, so that you can care for others, too) versus selfishness (the value judgment you or others level on yourself when you take time for yourself).

23. Take control of your mouth. Only you can control what goes into it, and what comes out!

24. Find something physical that you really love doing, and exercise regularly.

25. Check out your risk taking; psychologists say it's essential for growing holistically. How's your emotional, intellectual, social, spiritual, and physical risk taking?

26. Identify the stressors in your life and examine positive coping strategies to eliminate or reduce them.

27. Take credit where it's due in your life and take the blame when it's legitimate.

28. Daydream and be a dreamer. Recall the dreams/goals you had for yourself as a child or younger person and reflect on

what has happened to those childhood dreams.

29. Be content with who you are—change what you can, prevent what's preventable, and enjoy the rest.

30. Expect the best from yourself and others but remember that if you (or others) could be doing any better you (or they) would be.

31. Find something positive in all of your personal relationships and situations. Focus on and emphasize the positive even during the most trying circumstances.

32. Examine your attitudes toward change.

33. Develop the ability to bring out the best in others.

34. Look for the best in others and when you see it, tell them.

35. If you can't say something nice, don't say anything at all.

36. Sing out loud on the way to work.

✳ **To get even more out of this exercise, go back to each of the sentences you circled and think about them in more detail. Be specific about the changes you could make that would increase your self esteem or enhance your wellness. For example:**

#5. "Don't put yourself down," or #10: "Be gentle on yourself."

Don't get into the habit of putting yourself down or being unnecessarily critical of yourself. If you think like this, stop it. Criticism causes you to doubt yourself, decreases your self esteem, and erodes your spirit. Criticism rarely changes a thing. Pay attention to what you say to yourself, and when it's critical or negative, stop the thought and replace it with a more positive, affirming one. Work harder (yes, it's hard work to change a habit) to accept yourself and look for your strengths and the best you have to offer. When you affirm yourself, you have more ability and energy to invest in changes that can be positive and growth producing.

Pay attention to the fact that in the past you probably psychologically bought into and began believing these put downs about yourself to fulfill a need. I know this is a hard thing to accept. Tell yourself that at this point in time you need to find new and positive ways to fulfill your needs. Putting yourself down is an old negative pattern that you need to stop. (See the exercises "You Are What You Think" and "Negatrends.")

Another way to be gentle on yourself in addition to not putting yourself down, is to give yourself a gift: the gift of encouragement. Love yourself for who you are, not what you do, or how well you do it. "Just do it!" as Nike would say and do it now! Don't wait until you've lost the weight, are in a great relationship, or have advanced to a new position. Doesn't that sound like conditional love? "I'll love myself if I do this or I'm thus and so." Start now and be as loving and supportive to yourself as you can even though you're not a perfect individual with your act entirely together. Do you know anyone who is? If you don't know how to give yourself this kind of unconditional love and affirmation how can you possibly give or teach it to others?

#15: Form or join a support group.

A support group that focuses on specific issues is often very helpful. People who have been through a similar experience are often best equipped to offer direction and understanding.

Another way to 'support' yourself is to reach out to family or friends and allow them to help you. Try to be clear about what "helps." For example, you could ask people to listen attentively, ask you questions that help you understand the situation or your feelings. You could ask that they not pass judgment or take sides, and give you good counsel when, and if, you ask for it. Many people have been taught that it's a weakness to ask for support or help, but it takes courage and a strong individual to ask for help.

#11. Give yourself the gift of encouragement, support, and praise.

Learn to talk to yourself positively and praise yourself for who you are and what you do. Treat yourself with kindness, patience and tolerance to bring out the best in yourself. Chances are you'd do this for someone you love.

Scripture calls validation or encouragement a gift because it's unfortunately not the typical response we get from many people. It's actually easier for most people to criticize than it is to praise. Many of us criticize without even knowing it more frequently than praising or encouraging one another. Encouragement is the intentional opposite of criticism and comes in the form of being affirming or praising a person for a characteristic or accomplishment.

In addition, most of us have also have learned to accept criticism more readily than we accept praise. We've learned so many messages about criticism: "Turn the other cheek!," or "Let it roll off your back like water off a duck's back!" What about a new message which encourages you to refuse <u>uninvited criticism</u> in a way that is acceptable to you? For example, learn to say how you feel and what you want to change in the other person's behavior. "When you talk to me like that it makes me feel as if you're putting me down and sniping at me. If you have something to say to me that will help me, please talk to me in my office, not in front of other people in the halls." It's <u>direct</u>, <u>timely</u>, <u>authentic</u>, and <u>sets the boundaries</u> that you want the other person to respect. You also don't succumb to the temptation to put the other person down in return and escalate the situation.

Here are some personal wellness and self esteem ideas that caregivers from various professions who have been in my workshops have suggested:

- I try not to "should all over myself."

- I do more of what I want to do and not just what I should do.

- Intentionally day dream.

- Meet good friends for dinner.

- Call my "fan-club" friends for a pick me up.

- Turn off my beeper.

- Hire a housekeeper.

- I took time off to go to this self care seminar so I could get some ideas.

- Be more direct with my controlling boss.

- Consult with a nutritionist.

- Went back to school.

- I acknowledged that I am a "reforming perfectionist"! I do the best I can, but I don't let myself go nuts anymore when everything isn't perfect.

- I'm working at not feeling guilty for taking time off for myself. I'm a single mom.

- Go fishing. Alone, if I'm really strung out.

- I don't watch the news or read the paper for a while. Avoid negative people.

- Laugh out loud.

- Pay attention to looking my best instead of neglecting my appearance.

- Spend more time alone. When I'm alone, I don't beat myself up over being away from my other responsibilities.

- I spend a lot of time doing things to stay healthy but I'm still very stressed. I'm joining a support group.

- Reward myself or treat myself to something that pleases me.

- Get out into nature—I love to hike, fish, and camp.

- Attend seminars like this.

- Get a massage.

- Listen to relaxation tapes or good music.

♦ *Validation Envelopes* ♦

The need for self esteem is cogently expressed by the little boy who says:

> **"Mommy, let's play darts.**
> **I'll throw the darts and you say wonderful!"**

Are there any of us who don't want to feel good about ourselves and what we do? That's why this next exercise works so well.

Sincere praise or validation is a gift that encourages and inspirits a person. Everyone knows that a little encouragement goes a long way. But what we say needs to be something more than the same phrases used over and over. There are hundreds of affirmations you could share with your family, friends, colleagues, or children, no matter what their age. There are many words for it: praise, affirmation, positive regard, and validation. Scripture calls it the "gift of encouragement" and an encouraging word is a gift that helps us and others feel good about ourselves. Some people are naturally affirming; others can learn to be. Even Jesus Christ needed encouragement and one of his favorite disciples, Barnabus, gave him the gift. I figure if Christ needed encouragement, then we probably do too!

This exercise has it's roots in something we did as a family when our daughters were younger. It's a strategy I've introduced at workshops throughout the country that's a hit for people both at home and in the workplace!

You know that kids love mail, and no one, no matter what their age, outgrows the need for positive regard and sincere praise! Each of the members of our family would creatively decorate an envelope, put her or his name on the outside, and tape them to the refrigerator. My husband and I would jot our daughters and each other notes and put them in the validation envelopes. We encouraged them to do the same. The idea was to intentionally look for the best in each other, catch each other doing things well and right, and affirm the person for who they are as well as what they were doing.

The notes are short and simple and the intent of enhancing someone's self esteem or affirming them becomes a natural part of the relationships and a style of communication. Creating a nurturing family and loving relationships between siblings and with parents isn't something that "just happens" because you're related. Good relationships take time, effort, and consistent, positive communication. Here are just a few examples:

> *"Katie, I love your sensitivity and your hugs. I hope you never get too old to give, or receive, warm hugs!"*
>
> *"Kris, one of the things I love best about you is your determination! Keep up the good work! You can do anything you set your mind to!"*
>
> *"Tom, you're an incredible Dad—thanks for the ways you always encourage them! Someday they'll tell you themselves!*
>
> *"Nice going on that exam! Any chance all that intelligence is genetic? Can I catch some from you too?"*

It doesn't take a long time to jot someone an affirming note. In the process people learn about themselves through other people's eyes. There are daily opportunities to affirm someone and enhance someone's self esteem. Certainly one of the most significant gifts you can give your child as s/he matures is a healthy sense of self esteem and confidence.

There are a couple of secrets involved in giving the gift of encouragement though and they're simple:

- **Praise the person not just the performance**
- **Make your validation personal, specific, and sincere**
- **Praise in public if appropriate and remember that timing is everything**
- **Look for the characteristics or personal qualities you admire in the person, not just what the person does or accomplishes.**

Even an 'A' student can get a 'C', or an Olympic athlete can have an off day. We still all **need** and **deserve** validation no matter what our achievements are.

 You can adapt this strategy and use it at work with your colleagues as well. Get some plain, business-size envelopes and give one to each of your colleagues. Have each person write her/his name on the outside of the envelope and "decorate" it in any way that best represents them. Put the envelopes on the outside of your lockers or on a bulletin board where everyone has access to them.

Again, the purpose is simple: to build morale, team spirit, a positive workplace environment, share the gift of encouragement and to genuinely praise each other. Watch what happens when everyone adopts the attitude of "catching people doing something right" (instead of wrong). Encourage your peers to put a note of praise in each other's validation envelopes.

I know, you're probably thinking, "Listen, I don't have time to jot notes to my colleagues. I'm out straight and beyond busy!" But I'm not suggesting a dissertation here, just a short sentence or two that's intentionally shared to bring out the best in each other. It's true we're all busy, but, we all have 24 hours a day and how you utilize this time depends on your values. We all value colleagueship and a healthy working environment, but these don't materialize out of thin air! Here are a few examples:

"Congratulations! Con-grad-ulations! You're inspiring!"

"John, thanks for your ideas—as ever you're ahead of your time! You make me think!"

"You sure are one creative person! It's a pleasure working with you."

"Working with you is a treat, Danielle!"

"You must be proud of yourself for accomplishing that!"

"Connie, your caring counts!"

"Way to go! Always knew you could do it, Janine! You're so disciplined. I admire you."

"This is well written. You should submit it for publication."

Few of us want to feel poorly about ourselves so this strategy to enhance collegiality won't fail. Be creative and include physicians, social workers, dietitians and people from other departments in this strategy. Remind your colleagues that this is not a popularity contest. It's a simple, cost effective, creative way to bring out the best in each other.

◆ *Positive Regard, Public Praise, and Other Forms of Recognition* ◆

"There's only one thing worse than being talked about behind your back, and that's being ignored."
-Oliver Wendell Holmes

What's your initial reaction as you read this statement? Have either of these issues ever been your experience? Do you think it characterizes the experience many nurses have in their work environments?

Unfortunately both these issues, being talked about and not being validated, positively regarded, or publicly recognized enough, are frequently described by nurses no matter what their specialty or responsibilities. In some settings, (not where **you** work, of course!) there's too much back-stabbing and back-biting among nurses. The expression, "Nurses eat their young!" is familiar to many of us and was even the focus of a March, "Nursing 86" article by Judith Meissner.

Marie Manthey, a renowned nursing leader distributes buttons in her workshops. They have a cancellation sign drawn through 3 B's. She admonishes her colleagues to refuse to join in the "bitching, back-stabbing, and back-biting" that too often occurs.

Venner Farley, a wonderfully humorous and insightful nursing consultant appeals to nurses not to join the "BMW Club" which she says stands for "bitching, moaning and whining." It's true that complaining is sometimes an effective way to ventilate and deal with the stressors, but many people actually add to their own distress rather than relieve it when they complain too often.

A simple, but very effective way to deal with these types of negativity is to establish a ground rule of "no put downs." This includes everyone, no matter what their profession or position. You'll be surprised how often you'll notice the put downs, but with consistent reminders, people will begin to respond.

In addition to the stress that can result from interpersonal negativity and non-directed complaining, nurses do not get the recognition they deserve. They are the "Rodney Dangerfields" of health care and in spite of their significant and daily contributions and commitments, nurses go relatively unnoticed. It's in their absence that their presence is conspicuous and it's when caring is missing that it's noticed. Celebrating nurses and nursing once a year during Nurse's Week is not enough. What could be done on a more consistent basis that would be validating for nurses? What would be encouraging and serve as a pat on the back? What are some recognition strategies that are not merely limited to Nurses' Week?

Here are a few ideas I've introduced to hospitals and agencies throughout the United States that you can share. They are simple, cost effective strategies that increase the recognition caregivers richly deserve.

1.   In the lobby of the hospital, in addition to the pictures of the hospital administrators, why not put the pictures of nurses who should be recognized and honored for their excellence in caring? They could be displayed in a place where they are visible to the public. It sends a strong message that caring is valued and that the caregivers are the most valuable part of the hospital's or agency's resources. After all, the reason people must remain in the hospital is because they are in need of excellent nursing care. The art and science of nursing and the ethic of care needs to be more publicly affirmed and validated.

2.   What is one of the first things you notice in a physician's office? The diplomas, awards of recognition, certificates of achievement, and credentials, right? For most practitioners of nursing, the clinical area is their "office." Suggest that each nurse bring in her or his diplomas, certifications, and awards and put them on the walls throughout the unit. There they can be noticed by colleagues, families, and patients alike. The responses are overwhelmingly positive. Often we are unaware of the significant accomplishments, achievements, and amount of educational preparation that our colleagues have attained. In a large metropolitan hospital where I introduced this strategy, the compliments that were forthcoming and freely given served as a powerful image building as well as team building strategy. The pride and positive regard was evident.

3.   Validation Envelopes are an inexpensive way to acknowledge a colleague's value and contribution. The purpose of them is to affirm or validate your colleagues for not only certain behaviors and accomplishments, but also their character. Short notes dropped in someone's envelope serve to praise and validate in a way that even the spoken work cannot. See a more detailed discussion of this strategy in the previous exercise.

4.   One hospital has creative cards that anyone can be fill out for any employee. They call it the "ROSE" award. It stands for Recognition Of Service Excellence through Recognizing Our Special Employees. A rose is delivered to the nominated individual during the work day. It is seen as a special thank you, recognition of excellence in caring, or notable service and is highly valued. A short letter of appreciation or congratulations is also put in the person's employee file so that the recognition is noted in an official way and can be used during evaluation or for promotion.

      Recall some of the creative things you've seen done and think of some ways caregivers could appreciate each other, minimize compassion fatigue, and receive the recognition they deserve.

◆ *Validating One Liners* ◆

Sincerely praising or sharing an encouraging word is one way that caregivers can influence other colleague's or team's self esteem, help them continue to care effectively, or let them know you've noticed them or something they've done. An encouraging word is a gift that is inexpensive, yet priceless. It can help build an individual's morale and a team's effectiveness and increase satisfaction in nursing. It can help create a level of collegiality that's often elusive in a busy caregiving environment. Validation helps others feel better about themselves and at the same time enhances wellness in the workplace. Look for the best in your colleagues and validate them!

Think of some of the people you work with and some validating statements you'd be comfortable sharing with them. Jot the person's name down and something you could say to them that would be affirming in the spaces below.

1.

2.

3.

4.

5.

Catch people doing something right and look for the best in your colleagues. Don't let the characteristics of the person that make them special and the things people do go un-noticed or unappreciated.

 Attitudes are contagious — are yours worth catching?

◆ *Negative Self Talk* ◆

Negative self talk is often distorted, yet we begin believing the messages and start re-playing these tapes in our head. We must recognize the put downs or negative self talk and address them with more effective strategies.

Think of your own example and I'll share one of mine. Remember the negative voice or nitpicker inside your head relies on distortion and on you to listen and believe.

Let's say I've worked hard on an article for publication and it's been turned down. See if this internal dialogue sounds similar in style to the one's you have sometimes....

"I can't believe after all this work that this article isn't good. It's obviously poorly done. Other peers reviewed it and rejected it. It's awful." (*What am I doing in this internal dialogue? Looks like blowing things out of proportion to me.) And I have a way of doing that too often. How about you?*

"Was the "no" a final comment on my writing talents? Was the rejection letter publicized for the whole world to see?" (*A distortion*)

"Obviously your colleagues and the journal think you're a terrible writer." And this thought continues on to become "If this article was rejected, I must be a poor writer." (*An exaggeration*)

"I'm a failure." *I did realistically fall short on one of my goals. Does this discount all the other writing achievements? (More distorted thinking and exaggeration) Do I really think this? Then why do I tell myself such things? What good does it do me? Does it give me permission not to try again or not to enjoy past successes?*

"I always blow it when I really need to come through." (*More self flagellation*) "If I missed the mark this time, I must be slipping. But I do a lot of other things well most of the time. Writing is one aspect of the way I communicate." *This is a smaller voice, but it's there. When your heart speaks gently and tries to affirm you, listen. Its voice can get drowned out.*

"They don't think you're very talented, capable etc." *This is the final lie. Interesting. Now I'm reading other people's minds. Wow, I must be really talented! Can you see how distorted my internal dialogue became? What about yours?*

"I may not be the best writer, but I've had many articles that have been good and contributed new information. I am on to something that the literature doesn't discuss and it's even ahead of its time and proposes a very different point of view. I'm disciplined and I can improve it." *This is a more realistic and encouraging assessment of the situation and myself. It will allow me to stay focused on the task rather than wasting energy depreciating myself.*

Self esteem must come from real achievement, not just warm fuzzy validation and research shows that people need to feel successful about 75% of the time. It's fine to be sincerely validated by others, but positive regard also comes from affirming self talk or your own internal dialogue.

If you want to change your negative self talk pattern, here are some practical steps you can use:

- Pay attention to your self talk.
- Listen to what you are saying and identify it as harmful.
- Recognize negative self talk and self blame as self defeating.
- Make a decision to stop doing this to yourself.
- Get clear on what "messages" or "tapes" you choose to change and stop saying them as soon as you are aware of them.
- Clean up your self talk.
- Change the focus from what's wrong with you, to what you can do about the situation, or what's positive about you.

The more you respect yourself, the more you're able to learn about yourself and the world around you. Liking yourself is the bottom line for success in almost everything we do and the quality of our relationships.

✦ *I'm "Only" A Nurse!* ✦

"I'm only a nurse!" or "I'm just a nurse!" If I hear it again, I'll scream! So often it's the response I get when I ask, "What's your specialty?" or "What do you do?" I've been involved in nursing for almost 30 years and yet the answer has been surprisingly similar all this time.

Ask the same questions to physicians and listen to the responses. No matter how many times the question has been raised, I've never heard a physician respond, "I'm only a physician!" Never. I wonder why? What do you think? Does it have something to do with the way we socialize one another?

> *Nurses*
> *save lives*
> *touch deeply*
> *make a difference*
> *raise kids, inspirit elders*
> *perform the impossible*
> *balance, juggle*
> *write articles*
> *extend the gift of presence*
> *accomplish more with less each year*
> *conduct research*
> *present scholarly papers*
> *escort people into eternity*
> *counsel, comfort, heal*
> *soothe, care deeply*
> *earn many degrees including one in fine hearts*
> *have patience with patients*
> *are remarkable in a crisis*
> *take a lot of pressure*
> *have more than a job or career*
> *express commitment*
> *compassion, diligence, and*
> *are extra-ordinary and anything but average.*
> *—Diann Uustal*

Anyone who can handle and create all this is not "just'" or "only" a nurse! As the ANA slogan said a few years ago, "If you've got the brains, the patience, the heart, the courage, the commitment; be a nurse!" **Don't Put Yourself Down !**

♦ *"Negatrends"* ♦

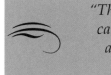 *"There is no value judgment more significant to one's psychological development and motivation than the estimate one passes on oneself."*
—*Nathanial Branden.*

What are some of the negative messages you say or "tapes" you play repeatedly to yourself? The fact is, if you talk negatively to yourself it creates a self-fulfilling prophecy and you become what you think. Why program your mind with disapproving thoughts which are so influential on your self esteem and your performance?

For example, a person might be saying: "I'm fat, I'm fat!" to herself when she looks in the mirror. And yet she'd like to lose weight. She's actually setting herself up for defeat by talking negatively to herself. People who really care about themselves don't put themselves down. It's like enlisting in an army against yourself. You'll change more quickly if you have respect for yourself and if you're encouraging. So instead of a put down, this woman could be saying: "I look and feel best when I weigh about 135 pounds." It's a radically different message than "I'm fat!" Or "I'm not as smart as so and so.," "I'm not as talented or creative" or whatever.

Recognizing the negative thought patterns and the negatrend this creates is the first step toward changing. This exercise will give you the chance to do this.

 Write some of the messages or "tapes" you play or negative one-liners you say to yourself:

1.

2.

3.

4.

5.

6.

Look at each of these put downs and examine them further by categorizing them. Use the designated letters to indicate the kind of put down you said to yourself and write them at the end of each sentence you wrote.

P **Physical**

Sp **Spiritual**

S **Social**

I **Intellectual**

E **Emotional**

Staying psychologically healthy involves countering the negative messages you say to yourself with positive self talk or messages. The first step is to **recognize** that you're putting yourself down, or "dumping" on yourself (you have heard of the "dumping syndrome" haven't you?). The second step is to **stop the behavior** which is probably a habit. The third is to **counter the put down with a more affirming statement.**

 Now take each of the put downs you identified and **think of what you could say to yourself that is positive.** If it was a physical put down, counter it with something you like about your physical self and so on. Write them in the space below.

1.

2.

3.

4.

5.

6.

By doing this, you are intentionally "re-programming" your mind to think more positively about yourself. I'm not saying to ignore something you want to change about yourself, I'm saying you will have more success and a healthier self esteem if you:

Here are some of the negative statements that have been shared by individuals in my workshops and seminars. Check those that are similar to what you've said to yourself.

○   "I'm not as smart, talented etc. as _____."

○   "I don't have any special abilities or talents."

○   "I'm too fat, not as attractive as, tall as. . ."

○   "Why bother! No one cares anyway!"

○   "I'm too old to change. I can't change after all these years."

○   "I'm too busy to take time for myself (or to exercise, eat right, etc)."

○   "It's the way I was raised. It's just the way I think."

○   "There's really not a whole lot I can do about it anyway, so I might as well just live with it."

•   Pay attention to the tenor of your internal dialogue. Are your comments typically about your physical or intellectual self, your emotional or social abilities, or your spiritual being?

•   In what area are you the most negative?

•   Is your dialogue with yourself about whether or not you're "worth" a particular effort or change?

♦ *You Are What You Think* ♦

Don't put yourself down. There are plenty of other people to do it for you!

Y ou'll see these statements a number of times in this book. Think about them and then use them as simple strategies for enhancing your wellness and self esteem.

Most of us are harder on ourselves than we need to be. Some of us fill our minds with negative self talk which erodes self esteem and robs us of confidence.

What are some of the "put downs" you typically say to yourself? Take a moment and jot them down in the space provided:

"Code"   Put Downs

_____   1.

_____   2.

_____   3.

_____   4.

_____   5.

_____   6.

 Look at the put downs you wrote on your list. Were they physical, emotional, social, intellectual or spiritual in nature? "Code" them by using the letter indicated for each category and write the letter(s) at the end of each of your responses.

P	Physical
E	Emotional
S	Social
I	Intellectual
Pr	Personality
T	Talent
C	Creativity
Sp	Spiritual

❋ Now take each of the put downs you identified and think of something you could say to yourself that is positive. For example, if it was a put down that involved your personality, counter with something you like about your personality. Write them in the space below.

1.

2.

3.

4.

5.

6.

Staying psychologically healthy involves countering the negative messages you say to yourself or get from others with positive messages or self talk.

Another thing that shapes your opinion of yourself is what other people say to you. These comments can be affirming or have a negative effect. For now, recall the negative messages and respond to the following questions:

- What are some of the negative messages you've heard from others?

- Are these messages the truth or is there some truth in them?

- Is the person who delivered the message frequently negative? Is this person typically a "put down artist?"

- Do you value this person's opinion?

- Should you pay attention to it more than what you feel about yourself?

- Did you invite the person to share the comments that were made?

- Does this person have your best interest in mind or is this a "hit and run" and you need to recognize that?

- What do you need to do, think, feel, or say in response to the comments made to you? Be specific and pay attention and practice your advice to yourself.

 Learn to say this wellness idea to yourself:
"No one can make you feel inferior
without your consent."
—*Eleanor Roosevelt*

◆ *Notes To Myself* ◆

*"If we monitored our own lives with the
intensity that we follow the stock market,
the sports page, or soap operas, we would be
witness to the most important drama of all."*
—Sid Simon

Journal writing is one of the ways to really take a closer look at who you are. How well do you know yourself? How much attention have you paid to the thoughts, habits, values and actions that come together to form the familiar patterns of your behavior?

A first step in discovering who you are is to systematically document and collect your thoughts. "Put it in writing" as AT&T would say. It's for your eyes only, unless you want to share it, so you can be free to explore anything you want to.

You could keep a special journal that helps you look back over various things in your life. This is actually the opposite of what a diary helps you do when you write about the here and now or the future.

Your journal could help you focus on your:
*Successes
Memorable moments, special occasions
Spiritual questions & insights
Value conflicts within yourself or with others
"Turning points" and the decisions you need to make
Affirmations people have shared with you
Questions you need to reflect on
"I'll never do that again!" journal
Ethical challenges
Hopes and goals
or anything that is of value to you...*

Here's something I wrote in my "Notes to Myself" journal. It's shared just to give you an idea of how short and simple an entry can be and yet how provocative and revealing it can be when you take the time for reflection.

Am I living in a way
which is deeply satisfying to me,
honors my potential,
truly allows me to express myself,
and share my gifts with others?

• Are you? If not, why not?

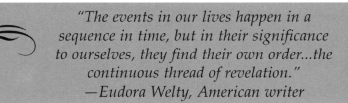

"The events in our lives happen in a
sequence in time, but in their significance
to ourselves, they find their own order...the
continuous thread of revelation."
—Eudora Welty, American writer

♦ *Cultivating Well Being* ♦

A positive mental attitude doesn't just "happen" for most people. Sometimes its a struggle to stay upbeat in the face of every day, real life difficulties and disappointments. For some individuals, a positive outlook just isn't their "style." And then there are others who always seem to be chipper and those who seem to "wear rose-colored glasses."

Stop and think about it for a minute. How do you frame your experiences? Are you a person who typically sees the day as "partially sunny" or "partially cloudy?" Is that water glass "half empty" or "half full"? Carl Rogers, a contemporary psychologist, calls this your "phenomenological field." How you typically "see" an event, the meaning you assign to it, and how you frame an experience is all part of this phenomenological field.

- What's your natural style?
- Can you do anything about it?
- Do you want to change it?
- Could the way you perceive things or respond to events be adding to your stress?
- Are there some attitudes you could intentionally learn to cultivate?

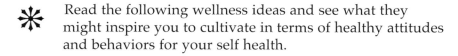 Read the following wellness ideas and see what they might inspire you to cultivate in terms of healthy attitudes and behaviors for your self health.

1.   Cultivate and nurture a positive mental attitude. For some of us this isn't so easy. Maybe you've wrestled with issues, struggled with past experiences, or it's just not your personality. So this wellness strategy will require commitment and discipline. Here's just one idea you could try that will influence your mental attitude. Foster an attitude of gratitude and express your feelings for the people and things you have in your life. Contentment isn't the ability to achieve what you want, but rather a response to what you have.

2. **Make balancing your life a priority**. New behavior patterns are hard to establish and stick with. Practice makes perfect, or at least improves your performance, so practice your balancing act in your personal, family and career life. Self discipline in areas that are hard to change requires a great deal of self control and clear goals. Celebrate the small successes you have frequently and you'll find your attitude about yourself, your abilities, and how you see other people will improve. There are many exercises in this book that will help you look at your balancing act. Don't forget that this balance should embrace a whole person perspective and include physical, emotional, intellectual, spiritual, and social components. If any component is neglected you run the risk of experiencing less balance and wellness in your life.

3. **Put someone in the "heart seat" each day.** (This is very different from the "hot seat") In other words, compliment them sincerely, jot them a short note of praise, FAX them an encouraging word, or pick up the phone and leave them a message of validation, not a request. It's encouraging to them and you'll feel good about taking the time to care. What goes around probably will come around and you'll profit twice!

By the way, you could put yourself in the heart-seat and gain immensely, too! This is also a good family meal-time strategy. Pick one of the members of your family and then have each at the table tell the individual in the heart seat what you love, appreciate or enjoy most about him/her. Watch what happens to his/her self esteem over time and the sense of safety, solidarity, and caring in your family. It works well with a caregiving team, too.

4. **Concentrate on what you like about yourself, the people in your life, your situation, career, and leisure activities**. This type of thought process tends to breed contentment rather than contempt. It's another way to cultivate that "attitude of gratitude."

5. **What do you want to be remembered for?** Try to lead your life I such a way that if you moved or weren't around more permanently, that people will remember certain qualities about you. If you had a nickname that you would want people to call you that describes how you'd like to be remembered? What would it be? We call one of my friends "Barney," not after the dinosaur the little kids love, but because John is an encourager by nature. Barnabus was the disciple who encouraged Christ and whose name meant "encouragement." So John is Barney to us. It describes him, the gift he brings, and how we know him and remember him best. Would the nickname that describes you be different for your personal and professional roles?

6.   Are you burned-up because you're burned out? Do you have a hard time saying no to all the personal and professional demands? Do you get angry with yourself and at others when you find yourself over committed? If you can't say "no," what's your "yes" going to be worth if you're spread too thin, tired, or ticked?

7.   Think about what was special about the day, what you did well, or what you learned while you're commuting home, during a "quiet time," or just before you fall asleep.
     Say to yourself: "It's hard to get through a day without:
          —being pleased about _____ .
          —learning something new.
          —being grateful to or for _____ .
Have some fun with your self talk and consciously appreciate yourself, those around you, and the good things about your life!

8.   Examine your patterns for relieving stress. Do you eat, drink alcohol, talk negatively to yourself, take your feelings out on others, smoke, or gamble when you're pressured? Are you creating more distress by the way you're responding to stress? Focus on one of your patterns and decide if and how you could change it to a healthier one.

9.   Identify and understand the real source of your anger.
A tremendous amount of emotional energy and time gets consumed by unresolved anger. There are many resources that can help you reflect on and plan strategies for more effectively dealing with your anger. Anger can reduce your quality of life. Unresolved anger can make you sick.

10.   Excellence is never an accident. When you see it in a person's character or accomplishments, or see it in yourself, take the time to validate it sincerely. You will appreciate the pat on the back and so will the other person. Don't let your own or someone else's capabilities go unnoticed.

11.   You are a human "being" not a human "doing." Give yourself some time just to "BE." How easy it is to confuse the essence of your worth if you base it only on what you do rather than who you are.

12.   Don't suffer from the "super person syndrome." Recognize that you are not superhuman, the fourth member of the Trinity, or whatever metaphor you like using. You have limits even when you refuse to recognize them. Tell yourself you're not striving for a confining notion of perfection, but rather to reach your own potential. Endeavor to do the best you can with the responsibilities and tasks that are important to you.

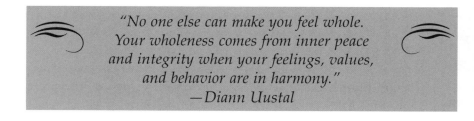

"No one else can make you feel whole.
Your wholeness comes from inner peace
and integrity when your feelings, values,
and behavior are in harmony."
—Diann Uustal

◆ *Wellness "Indicators"* ◆

There are a variety of indicators that reveal your state of wellness. Some of them are feelings or experiences, others a state of mind or spiritual. Check the items below that you think are indicators of your state of wellness.

_____ I am more able to enjoy the here and now.

_____ I am less critical of myself.

_____ I have more energy to praise, validate and encourage others.

_____ I am less judgmental of others.

_____ I feel happy inside.

_____ I am a more calm and peaceful person.

_____ I "stay in the room" more often and concentrate on the here-and-now, not the past or future.

_____ I am less interested in what others think and in pleasing them.

_____ I am more lighthearted and smile and laugh more.

_____ I allow things to develop and happen rather than always trying to plan them out and orchestrate them.

_____ I have lowered my expectations of perfection in terms of how I should perform or others should behave.

_____ I feel closer to people in my family and my friends.

_____ I count my blessings more often than focusing on what's wrong or missing.

_____ I can find something good in difficult or bad situations more easily.

❋ What are some indications of your wellness that you're aware of that weren't included above? Write your responses in the spaces below:

1.

2.

3.

4.

5.

♦ *Balcony People* ♦

When you hear the term "life support" how many of us think of the <u>people</u> in our lives as our life support system? Think of the folks who have influenced your life positively as your "Balcony People." These are the people in your personal life or those who you know from your professional experiences that root for you and cheer you on and up! Read the descriptions of some of the things that these people might do or offer you and jot the person(s) name who does this in the spaces provided. You can use a person's name more than once. It can be someone you know intimately or a person you've never even met. Turn to the people in your balcony and ask for their support when you need it.

Balcony People Who:		Personally	Professionally
1.	Support me	1.	1.
2.	Stimulate/challenge me	2.	2.
3.	Make me laugh	3.	3.
4.	Energize me	4.	4.
5.	Make me feel good about myself	5.	5.
6.	I am totally comfortable with	6.	6.
7.	Accept me unconditionally	7.	7.
8.	I go to when I'm down	8.	8.
9.	Praise, validate and affirm me	9.	9.
10.	Have influenced me the most	10.	10.
11.	I can tell anything to	11.	11.
12.	Admire me	13.	13.
13.	I trust implicitly	14.	14
14.	I can be spontaneous with	15.	15.

◆ *The Ties That Bind* ◆

Good relationships don't just happen. They're created.
Whether it's a friendship, a marriage, relationships with
your children or co-workers, there's energy and effort required to
make them qualitative and to nurture, protect, and enhance
them.

Think about your personal or professional relationships.
What are you doing to enrich the relationship with your hus-
band/wife, children, or friends? What are you doing to enhance
collegiality where you work?

1.   Things you've done:

2.   Things you typically do:

3.   Things you could do more of:

4.   Things you could do less of:

5.   Ideas you've heard about that might work for you:

6.   Some things you'd like the other person to do:

7.   The gifts you bring to the relationship:

8.   The benefits you receive:

9.   What are the "ties that bind"(events, characteristics, memories) your relationship over time?

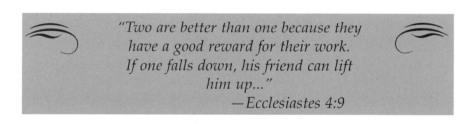

"Two are better than one because they have a good reward for their work. If one falls down, his friend can lift him up..."
—*Ecclesiastes 4:9*

◆ *Basement People* ◆

U nfortunately there are also "basement" people in our lives. You know, the ones that seem to get to you faster than anyone else on the planet! Perhaps you call them "vacuum cleaners" or "toxic," but we all have a few.

Maybe they're like that because they've had some tough times and are hurting. Possibly they don't know how negative they sound because few people tell them. Conceivably they might not know how to break out of an old pattern. Then again, some basement people are "negaholics" and are "addicted" to their style and don't want to change. **The fact is, they wear you out no matter what the reason.** Perhaps they're people you work with on a daily basis or a part of your family, so what can you do?

There are lots of strategies to be sure. One positive one is to try **"creative neglect."** Since you will probably have continued contact with some basement people, try **limiting the times** or **timing** of your interaction to correspond with your energy as well as your obligations. For example, you could call this particular person only when you're feeling **rested up** enough to listen or when you've got **enough energy** to tolerate the negativity that may be directed at you. Both these responses are examples of "creative neglect." **It's not your typical response**, but it is a strategy you can use to help you take care of yourself and meet your own needs when you know it's necessary.

You must also recognize that **"constructive criticism"** is really **"constrictive cruticism"** and is most likely a product of the other person's agenda and material. Another part of a healthy strategy is to identify who these "basement people" are and how to respond to them in more proactive ways when the negative criticism is directed at you.

In the space below list some of the "basement" people you deal with in your personal and professional life.

1.   4.

2.   5.

3.   6.

What are the things they **typically say or do** that are negative, critical or wearing on you?

1.

2.

3.

4.

5.

What are some **responses you could make** to each of the individuals you have identified when they are unnecessarily negative or critical?

1.

2.

3.

4.

5.

If you were able to respond to them in these ways, **do you think it would improve the relationship** or get them to be less critical? Why or why not?

What other strategies could you use to effectively and proactively deal with the basement or toxic people in your life? Be as specific as you can and identify a few of your ideas here.

1.

2.

3.

4.

5.

Could one of your strategies be that you forgive them and get on with your life and direct your attention to more important goals?

•   What would it take for you to really do this?

•   What would your decision to forgive them enable you to do differently?

•   How would it change you?

•   How would it change your perceptions of the situation?

•   Do you think it would it change you or the other person more?

•   How difficult is this part of the strategy regarding forgetting, forgiving, and moving on?

♦ *Dealing With Vultures, Basement People, And Vacuum Cleaners* ♦

Now let's talk about the put downs that come from other people. What do "vultures", "basement people", and "vacuum cleaners" have in common? No this isn't a joke. It's no laughing matter! What they all have in common is that they put people down and they're good at it. Have you ever noticed how some people use humor to mask a put down? It might get a laugh, but it's usually at someone's expense and it's still a put down. These types of people seem to delight in needling others or always have something off color or critical to say. Let's face it, their behavior is toxic!

We all have them! Maybe you call them put down artists or vultures as Sid Simon would say. I call them toxic, or basement people (a sharp contrast to balcony people) or vacuum cleaners. They seem to suck the life force right out of you with their negativity faster than most of the other people on the planet! They can "get to you" faster than anyone else and know just how to "yank your chain"!

So how do you respond to these put down artists? Few of us get formal instruction or practice in self esteem in the classroom. Instead we learn the capitals of the states, but don't know how damaging it is to put others down or to listen to the put downs. Nor are we taught any strategies to deal with put downs once they occur.

What are some of the negative messages or put downs you've heard from others or "tapes" you've learned to play? **Come on, write them here even if it makes you squirm a bit. (You could even write the person's name next to the statement.)**

1.

2.

3.

4.

5.

Now that you've written some of them down, here's something we should all have been taught in school. It's a simple wellness concept:

Get off my foot!

Sometimes people need to be told "Stop, that hurts my feelings! Especially when you say it in front of other people! If you have something to say to me that will help me grow, fine, say it to me in private. Otherwise keep your negative opinions to yourself!" You need to develop some ways to deal with the put down artists. Go ahead, think of some "one-liners" that you can rehearse and have ready if this person has another put down. Write them next to the numbers that correspond to the messages and names you just identified.

Another wellness strategy might be to use a technique I call "de-fusing." You do this when you take a value-judgment someone else says about you and make it more positive. For example: "You're so stubborn." Stubborn sounds negative to most of us. So "de-fuse" the message. "Connie, I'm so glad you noticed!" (This is validation and you probably have her attention now). "I am persistent..." (this is the "de-fusing." "Persistent" is a more positive value judgment than "stubborn"). Perhaps if you've been thinking how to deal with this situation for a while, you'll be able to finish the conversation with "...especially when I'm right!"

Now for some of us this may be a bit much, but you did not resort to putting the other person down, and it allowed you to walk away intact and perhaps with a message left behind that indicates you don't want to be put down.

 "The single most important cause of your success or failure has to do with what you think of yourself."
—*Nathaniel Brandon*

♦ *"Constructive Criticism"*
or
"Constrictive Cructicism"? ♦

A long time ago I learned about "constructive" criticism from Sid Simon, my mentor, dissertation chairperson, and now lifetime friend. Actually Sid learned it from a wise, older school teacher, Mamie Porter, but that's another story.

Sid and Mamie have got me believing that very little criticism is truly "constructive." They say most of it is negative criticism and they call it "constrictive cruticism." Maybe it's the way it's communicated and the fact that it may damage more than help. Perhaps it's even the other person's "agenda" and has little to do with helpful approaches for the receiving party's benefit.

I think criticism can be constructive when it's in our best interest and when the party delivering the message does so with kindness and respect. You know the difference right away. For most of us it's an intuitive thing. The point is most of us are far too willing to criticize and much slower to praise. This goes for the way we treat ourselves as well as others.

If it will help, think of certain relationships you have and particular situations. For example, the dinner table with your children, evaluation reviews with colleagues, conversations on the phone about someone else. You know how it starts or maybe you've said:

> **"It really bothers me to tell you this but..."**
> **"I know it's none of my business, but..."**
> **"You've been doing a good job, but..."**
> **"I know this will bother you worse than it does me, but..."**

Stop, look at the word "but," and listen to the things you or others are saying.

What are some things we can do to help us to "hold our tongue" or "reign in the criticism" others may experience as constrictive? Here are some reminders for you to use, or for you to teach others to use, before any of us criticize. Try to run through these reminders before you give yourself permission to criticize.

1. First, remember most people need more praise and less criticism.

2. Second, cultivate the attitude that most people are probably doing the best they can. If they could be doing any better, they would be. If they're not, and this is always a value judgment (yours), then proceed.

3. Third, consider if you really do have this person's best interests, growth and development at heart.

If you've considered these three things, then ask yourself:

- Is there a **trust** relationship here? Does this person have this type of relationship with me or I with her/him?

- Was I **invited** to share my "constructive" thoughts and opinions? Is it part of my role or relationship with them to offer appraisal? (for example, your children, employees) If it isn't part of your relationship, then you weren't "invited."

- Is this person in any shape to hear it? **Timing** is everything. Is this a good time or is it insensitive?

- Can they **"hear"** what you are saying? We're talking psychological hearing and openness. Will they "allow" you to be the messenger?

- Have they **heard it before**? And again, and again.....

- Can they **do anything about it**?

- Are they really in need of **more validation** and **affirmation rather than criticism**?

- **Is this your "material" or "agenda"?** How much of what you want is what is motivating you to say something?

- Is your commitment or relationship deep enough to stick around and **pick up the pieces** if your criticism hurts. Or is it just a **"hit & run"**?

Hopefully these reminders are helpful to you. I'm not saying that we don't have the right and responsibility to appraise each other's behavior at times. I'm talking about people who seem to be too quick with criticism that's negative. This kind of "constructive criticism" colors a person's self esteem gray. Maybe along with these reminders it's also good to recall what we read in Bambi when Thumper's mother taught Thumper:

"If you can't say something nice, don't say it at all!"

 If you are the receiver of some unsolicited "constructive criticism" you may want to consider the following questions before you take the criticism to heart...

- Is it the truth or is there some truth in it?

- Is the person often negative or having a bad day? Is this person typically a put down artist?

- Do you value this person's opinion?

- Should you pay attention to it more than what you feel about yourself?

- Did you invite the person to share his/her comments with you?

- Does this person have your best interest in mind or is this a "hit and run" and you need to recognize that?

- What do you need to do, think, feel or say in response to the comments made to you?

"Keep the other person's well being in mind when you feel an attack of soul purging truth coming on."
—Betty White, American actress

♦ *A Person Learns What They Live* ♦

A person who lives with criticism,
learns to condemn.
A person who lives with hostility,
learns to fight.
A person who lives with ridicule,
learns to be shy.
A person who lives with shame,
learns to feel guilty.
A person who lives with tolerance,
learns to be patient.
A person who lives with encouragement,
learns confidence.
A person who lives with praise,
learns to appreciate.
A person who lives with fairness,
learns justice.
A person who lives with security,
learns to have faith.
A person who lives with approval,
learns to like her/himself.
A person who lives with acceptance and friendship,
learns to find satisfaction in life.

— Author Unknown

Adapted from the poem "Children Learn What They Live."

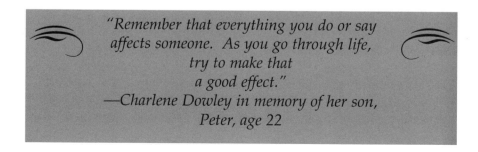

"Remember that everything you do or say
affects someone. As you go through life,
try to make that
a good effect."
—Charlene Dowley in memory of her son,
Peter, age 22

♦ *Ways To "Take Care"* ♦

Here are some apparently easy ways to "take care" that have been shared by caregivers participating in my workshops. Check off the ideas that could help you take care of yourself more effectively and enhance your quality of life:

☐ I live my life in such a way that I have few regrets.

☐ I am the author of my life. I can "edit" many circumstances easily, others are more difficult to understand and change.

☐ I try not have a lot of "unfinished business" in my relation-ships.

☐ I like to be as consistent as I can between what I say I value and what I do.

☐ I don't "catastrophize" during a tough time. I try not to make things worse than they are by over-dramatizing them.

☐ I take one day at a time and stay in the present.

☐ I break what's difficult into more manageable parts and feel good about what I accomplished along the way.

☐ I count my blessings, not focus on my problems when I'm feeling down or pressured. This isn't as easy as you think.

☐ I work at creating the attitude that "everything can work together for good" even when it doesn't seem that way. I intentionally choose to believe that there's a silver lining in a dark cloud.

☐ I try not to let myself waste time and energy on worrying about things I can't change or have little control over. I spend more energy on changing the things I can change.

☐ I have learned the longer I carry my problem around alone, the heavier it gets. Two are better than one. Sharing my issue helps.

☐ I don't take myself or the work I do too seriously.

☐ I try to cultivate health, hope and happiness. I do more than wish upon a star, it's hard work.

☐ I don't feel guilty for trying to take care of myself. When I do, I'm a whole lot nicer to the people who count in my life and a lot more peaceful inside.

☐ A long time ago, I decided it's never too late in terms of relationships. Never too late to say something special, to ask for forgiveness, or to take a risk.

☐ I've found a little love goes a long way—a lot goes even further. I invest wholeheartedly in my relationships.

☐ I constantly remind myself to put first things first in my life and to stay focused on my priorities. When situations are demanding I need more strength and discipline to accomplish this, but "first things first" is a good metaphor for me.

♦ S - T - R - E - S - S ♦

Life and living can be stressful.
"Can be!" you snicker! "It is stressful!"

As a caregiver you know this all too well. The demands of personal and professional commitments sometimes combine to form a fast paced, no time for yourself lifestyle that leaves you whipped and feeling stretched.

Simply defined, stress is any physical or emotional change. The noted researcher, Hans Selye defined stress as "a recurring imbalance resulting in daily wear and tear on the body that leads to dysfunction and debilitation." Enough stress over time can lead to social, emotional or physical problems and be severe.

Change can be either positive or negative. An example of eustress, or positive stress, could be a career promotion or a move to a new house. They are seen as positive, but still involve change and stress. Negative stress, or distress, occurs because of the death of someone you love, being injured, or changing positions because of "right-sizing."

What are some positive and negative stressors you've experienced in the past six months?

Positive Stressors	Negative Stressors
•	•
•	•
•	•
•	•
•	•

Stress can also be chronic or acute. Getting caught up in traffic (directly proportional to how late you are for an appointment), the button falling off the blouse that goes best with your suit, or dealing with toxic people in your life are examples of the chronic, everyday stressors that can wear us out. By themselves, they aren't such a big deal. It's when they all seem to happen at the same time or we don't take time to manage them that they get out of proportion.

Acute stress is the kind of flight or fight reaction you experience when confronted with a threat where you need to react quickly. Slamming on the breaks because of an animal darting in front of your car is one example. Your body gets ready for action by increasing the heart and respiratory rate, your pupils dilate, other senses become more keen, blood flow is shunted to the muscles, blood sugar rises, and the pituitary releases hormones like adrenaline. Shortly after this response you feel shaky or maybe tired and you experience the toll this type of stress exacts from the body.

Stress is derived from two sources: external/environmental or internal/emotional. Disturbing sounds, a smoke filled room, or demanding individuals are external stressors. Internal sources of stress arise from one's own thought processes about how well a particular task should be done or what will happen if certain things don't take place.

It's fine to have a cognitive understanding about stress; however, it's quite another matter to take the appropriate steps to temper its effects on our lives.

 Take the next few minutes to think about the things you experience as stressors in your life.

- **What are the things that usually bother you or get to you? Jot them down here:**

- How do you typically react to things that cause you stress?
    —Do you get angry quickly?
    —Or do you keep a lid on your feelings until you can't control them any more and then blow up?
    —Do you use substances to control your feelings?
    —Do you call a friend or go for a walk? What's your typical response? Write a few of them down:

Everyone responds to stress differently. Some of us are better at it than others. Some of us could improve our health if we utilized more effective strategies for dealing with the pressures of life.

• Where do you register or carry your stress in your body? Do you have a stiff neck or back, develop migraines, ulcers ?

• How do you respond to stress emotionally? With feelings of anger, depression, or frustration?

• What happens to you spiritually when you're under a lot of stress? Is your faith or other expressions of your spirituality a first resort or a last resort?

• How does stress affect you intellectually?

• When you're feeling stressed, in general, are you the kind of person who wants to be around people or be alone? Is your typical response your best strategy?

  By identifying what causes you stress and planning for how you can deal with it, you have taken two essential steps in beginning to manage your stress more effectively.

✦ *Recognizing When It's All Too Much* ✦

The term "burnout" is a familiar one. One of my friends says in a cavalier fashion that she'd "...rather burn out than rust out!" I agree, but either can be harmful. The fact is some of us have a hard time recognizing and then admitting when the demands in our lives need adjusting in relation to the relaxing and recovery times.

• What if you've had enough and you **refuse to admit it?**

• Or what if you're badly **in need of a respite, but can't get it?**

• What if you been giving yourself so little slack for so long now that's it's just a **bad habit** and you **don't even recognize it?**

Any one of these situations can cause any of us to "burnout." It happens when there are too many demands and too little time or ability to refuel. Typically we get angry at the people or situations that demand more from us than we can give. You can make it on "faith and fumes" once in a while, but a lifestyle like this will result in burnout. You, too may be saying I'd rather burnout than rust out, but anyone who's crashed and burned can tell you that being consumed by the fire isn't fun and the rehabilitation is no picnic either!

So what do you do then? Here are some approaches and suggestions that could help you prevent or limit burnout or rebalance a demanding lifestyle:

Acknowledge your experiences and feelings. Tell others you are experiencing stress, anxiety, or unhappiness.

Pay attention to what causes you stress. Keep a journal. When you feel tense, what happens? What helps?

Develop some strategies to decrease or eliminate the stressor(s). For example, ask people you trust how they deal with various stressors. Get some "ventilatory support" and talk out your feelings.

Find some things that make you feel good while you're going through the tough times. Psychologists tell us that doing something we enjoy and doing something that helps others are the two most significant ways to control stress.

Move! In other words, exercise or do something physical that will help your body release it's natural endorphins or mood elevating chemicals.

Get involved in a support group or supportive community of people who are dealing with similar issues where you can share strategies for coping and tell your story.

Seek counseling or outside professional help.

Make sure there are no other causes, such as a physical ailment or undiagnosed illness, that could be contributing to your stress.

Care for the whole of you. You have physical, emotional, social, spiritual, and intellectual components that make up who you are. Neglecting any one of these areas means you could be out of balance with your self care.

 Create a quiet place in your home...at work...in your heart...where you can go for peace and re-creation.

◆ *Self Imposed Stressors?* ◆

We all realize that life can be stressful, more so some days than others. Some careers and jobs are more taxing than others. However, some of the stressors in our lives are self-imposed and some come from our *perceptions of situations and people* and therefore can be reduced or eliminated by relearning a new pattern of response.

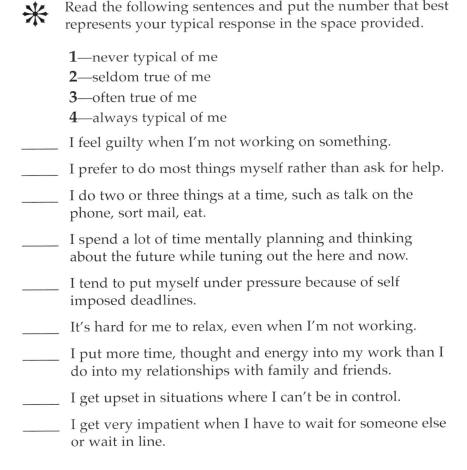

Read the following sentences and put the number that best represents your typical response in the space provided.

    1—never typical of me
    2—seldom true of me
    3—often true of me
    4—always typical of me

_____ I feel guilty when I'm not working on something.

_____ I prefer to do most things myself rather than ask for help.

_____ I do two or three things at a time, such as talk on the phone, sort mail, eat.

_____ I spend a lot of time mentally planning and thinking about the future while tuning out the here and now.

_____ I tend to put myself under pressure because of self imposed deadlines.

_____ It's hard for me to relax, even when I'm not working.

_____ I put more time, thought and energy into my work than I do into my relationships with family and friends.

_____ I get upset in situations where I can't be in control.

_____ I get very impatient when I have to wait for someone else or wait in line.

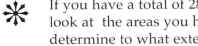

If you have a total of 28 points or higher, you may want to look at the areas you have marked with a 3 or 4 and determine to what extent they are signs of workaholism and sources of stress in your life.

Can you deal with the stressors more effectively? Many times your patterns of predictable responses can throw you off balance. Too often they are *habits or responses* that increase your stress and *need to be unlearned.* By identifying these situations, recognizing your typical responses to them, and then determining what you can do differently, you will have more energy to devote to other activities.

In the space below, jot down what you can do specifically to reduce this stressor. Identify if it is self imposed or not.

Identify the person(s) or situation(s) in which you learned this pattern or the person(s) from whom you learned this response pattern.

The Situation   **My Typical Response**
1.
2.
3.
4.

What I Can Do Differently to Reduce the Stressor
1.
2.
3.
4.

 Ways you can learn more from this strategy:
•   Identify additional stressors and your responses and write them down. Categorize your response by using the numbers provided.
•   Indicate in writing what you can and cannot do to reduce these stressors in your life.
•   Talk to other individuals you know personally and professionally and learn from them.

Listen to some of the statements about what's stressful for them that participants have shared in my workshops. Do any of them sound familiar?

"I have to change the notion that I am my work."

"I have to stop believing that when I get antsy, I should get up and start working on one of 50 projects that are available to me..."

"Adrenaline is just as addictive as other substances like alcohol and drugs, but I've found it a lot more handy. And meditation was a fix for me so I could continue to practice my addiction."

"Hard work, a valued skill as a child, may be killing me now. I am busy beyond what time allows and I have to change this."

"I decided being too tired on weekends to have fun was a symptom of doing too much during the week."

"When I fill my calendar, I don't have time to do the things I want to do for myself."

A workaholic culture makes it easy to use work as a temporary fix to avoid dealing with certain problems.

 If workaholism is the addiction of choice for the unworthy, how does one get worthy?

♦ *"Mini-Vacations:"Taking A Daily Time Out From Stress* ♦

W hy is it that we wait until we go on vacation at appointed times of the year to relax and unwind? Sure it's easier when you're removed from the daily demands of family or career to pamper yourself, but a more effective wellness strategy is to take some time out during each day to consciously relax and control stress. I'm not talking only at the end of the day. Some of us might even be doing that pretty well. I'm thinking more of frequent mini-breaks during the day to help control the build up of stress. It will help you cope more easily with the pressures you experience. Here are some ideas:

○   It can be as simple as closing your eyes for even as little as 30 seconds to a minute and taking a few, slow, deep breaths and thinking only of something relaxing. Why don't you stop what you're doing right now and take a few deep breaths?

○   You could sit comfortably, close your eyes, and think about a person in your life who adds to your quality of life. Imagine them sitting across from you and what you would say to them about how they enrich your life. At some point you might want to pick up the phone and share what you were thinking and feeling, send a card, or let them know face-to-face if possible.

○   You could sit or lie down for five minutes and tense and relax your muscles and imagine yourself in a very peaceful situation or beautiful location like sitting on the beach and watching the sun set slowly into the ocean.

The point is, if you do this as frequently as three or four times a day, these mini vacations will do wonders for your overall mental and physical health. You might be saying, "Oh sure, with my schedule (or my kids, or my job) there's no time for something like this!"

Are these reasons or excuses?

- No time? *We all have 24 hours a day. How you spend your time is based on what you value.*

- You hear a lot about taking responsibility for your own health. *No one else can help you take care.*

- What is the price you'll pay if you don't take some time out? *Can you afford not to take time out?*

- How do you feel when you're not on so much of a treadmill that you're not able to enjoy your life?
    - What's it like when you step back off that pace just a bit?
    - Do you relate to others better?
    - Are you happier?
    - Are you more gentle on yourself?

Think about these questions. Then take whatever action will give you a mini vacation and is in your best interest.

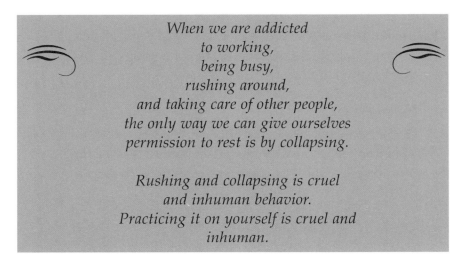

*When we are addicted
to working,
being busy,
rushing around,
and taking care of other people,
the only way we can give ourselves
permission to rest is by collapsing.*

*Rushing and collapsing is cruel
and inhuman behavior.
Practicing it on yourself is cruel and
inhuman.*

◆ *Personal Strategies for High Level Wellness and Stress Control* ◆

Each of us pays attention to our wellness and handles stress differently. Even what causes us to feel better or experience stress is different. There's no one right or best way to create more wellness in your life from a holistic perspective or to handle stress more effectively; however, not to use some simple, effective strategies can be detrimental to your overall health in the long run.

We all know that each one of these suggestions are easier said than done. Change is difficult at best, but you could use each of the suggestions as a strategy or "care plan" by first recognizing it's importance to you and then identifying specifically how you could use it in your everyday life. Read through the proposals and then decide which would be beneficial for you. Then make sure you follow through. That's the hardest part. We all know what we could or "should" do, but then we don't act on what we know would be good for us.

PHYSICAL/PHYSIOLOGICAL:

1.   Get regular physical exercise. Do something you love to do. Vary your activities or "cross train."

2.   Practice techniques that help you relax and unwind.

3.   Intentionally breathe deeply to relieve stress.

4.   Eat a balanced diet, drink at least six glasses of water a day and don't skip meals to decrease calories.

5.   Try to spend some of your time outside each day. Eat your lunch outside if possible.

6.   Pay attention to the harmful substances you use and decrease or eliminate their use.

7.   Seek preventative or restorative professional help earlier rather than later.

8.   Take a quick walk. It's one of the best ways to revitalize your body and mind. If you can't do this, at least walk a few flights of stairs to change your pace or help relieve stress.

EMOTIONAL:
1. Alter your emotional climate when you need to. Intentionally laugh, sing, or smile to lift your spirits.
2. Have a healthy sense of regard and respect for yourself. Share this attitude with and toward others.
3. Be realistic about what you expect whether it's your fears, or goals and dreams.
4. Reduce your worrying by being clear about the difference between what you can control what you can't.
5. Reduce the number of changes in your life.
6. Reduce the number of time oriented pressures in your life.
7. Talk out your feelings and try not to hide your feelings.
8. Discipline yourself to think and say positive things if you tend to be critical.
9. Examine the company you keep. Think about the people you're around, the TV you watch, music you listen to and how these things influence your feelings, mood and behavior.
10. Learn to make the hard decisions in your life with more confidence and peace.
11. Walk away from the problem. Sometimes this is the most sensible thing to do. Removing yourself from a situation for a few minutes or for longer may allow you to reflect on the situation better and choose a strategy for addressing it. If you find yourself doing this too often, you will want to look at other ways of dealing with the situation.

PSYCHOSOCIAL:
1. Simplify your lifestyle.
2. Help others and see what happens to you.
3. Set standards for yourself and live up to your own potential. "Compete" with yourself not with others.
4. Express your creativity. Develop hobbies or interests that are fulfilling to you.
5. Spend some free time with "support" groups. This could be a gourmet group or a discussion group.
6. Know "when to say when" and when you've had enough. Give yourself permission to quit.

7. Choose your priorities: You can't do everything you'd like to do in the course of the day, so set your priorities. Must do, would like to do, if there's time to do. Be satisfied with and tally up your accomplishments instead of being frustrated by your failures.

SPIRITUAL:

1. Develop an attitude of praise and gratitude.

2. Be an encourager to yourself and others. Look for the best in yourself and others and compliment them sincerely. Catch people doing things right.

3. Stay close to your values and try to walk them as well as talk them.

4. Ask for forgiveness. Accept it. Give it freely. Forgive and forget or at least get on with your life.

5. Be humble.

6. Find out what's your "soul work." Do something that allows you to use your time and talents in ways that others can benefit from. You'll benefit too.

7. Find a community of people who believe as you do and who are growing spiritually.

8. Get to know the individual you call God and make up your mind to invest in the relationship. You can't get to know someone without spending time with the person and it's true in a spiritual relationship too.

9. Decide which resources about your faith you need to consult and learn from. Study and learn and test yourself.

"I long to put the experiences of fifty years at once into your young lives, to give you at once the key to that treasure chamber, every gem of which has cost me tears and struggles and prayers, but you must work for these inward treasures yourselves."
—*Harriet Beecher Stowe*

◆ *Common Sense For A Healthy Self* ◆

As professionals we're always coordinating and orchestrating the care of others, so it should be simple to create a care plan for ourselves, right? Perhaps these ideas will seem like common sense. But you know what they say about common sense. It's not so common!

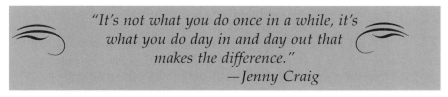

> *"It's not what you do once in a while, it's what you do day in and day out that makes the difference."*
> —*Jenny Craig*

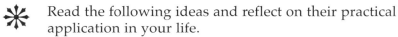 Read the following ideas and reflect on their practical application in your life.

1.   Taking personal responsibility for your health physically, emotionally, intellectually, socially, and spiritually is not easy, but it's the first step. Like it or not, there's no one who can do a better job at taking care of yourself than you. Besides, it's your health and your responsibility.

2.   Start today with the changes you know are healthful. Make your choices one meal at a time or for one day at a time. Don't beat yourself up if you don't always stick to the care plan.

3.   Balance. We all know life can be more challenging some days or years than others. Try to stay in balance from a holistic perspective. What this is and means is different to each one of us. It's also different for the same person as life continues to unfold.

4.   Increase your happiness quotient. Identify the things that bring you happiness and joy and enhance your quality of life. Give yourself a "homework assignment" and try to do at least something pleasurable or satisfying each day. This will result in benefits for you and the people around you.

5.   Identify and decrease the stressors in your personal and professional life. Identify the stressors and pay attention to your reactions. Develop strategies for decreasing the overall level of stress in your life. Some situations and habits can be corrected easily, others will take a real commitment and time to change.

6.   Make sure your goals and expectations are realistic. The best way to defeat yourself is to establish a goal that is unreachable because it's unrealistic, too lofty, there's too little time, or it requires more than you are able to invest. Maybe it's not even what you want and it's someone else's goal for you. Your goals should be measurable, manageable, and meaningful to you.

7.   Give yourself permission to relax and take some time for yourself each day. Learn to take "mental health breaks" or "mini-vacations" even if they are only for 15 minutes at first. Discipline yourself not to think of all the things that you should be doing while you're on your break. Enjoy the time as completely as you can so you can go back to what you were doing refreshed.

8.   Prioritize your commitments based on your values. The ones that are probably the most precious to you involve relationships that have stability and meaning over time. Many of us do not give appropriate time and attention to the relationships that are the most significant even though we say they count the most.

9.   Learn to say "no" if you are pressured and over committed. Practice if you have to. Be clear about what you really can say no to and stick to your decision. Learn to say no without feeling guilty. Practice thinking that every problem is not your sole responsibility.

10.   Treat yourself like you treat your best friend. Think of your best friend and how you enjoy doing something to show you care for him or her. Now do something special for you and "be-friend" yourself.

11.   Be a person of encouragement—to yourself. Clean up your self talk and be as affirming to yourself as you are with people you really care about. Don't "dump" on yourself or put yourself down.
12.   Make your physical fitness a priority. We're not talking about being an Olympian here, but rather being committed to a

balanced fitness program that includes stretching, aerobic exercise, and strength exercises. "Cross train" and participate in a number of different sports for the fun of it. A great way to stay in shape is to "sneak" exercise into your life! Walk or ride a bike instead of drive, park further away, use the stairs instead of the elevator, and if it's available take advantage of the medical center's walking paths or track on the roof for a break to clear you mind. Research shows if you start a fitness program with a friend you are more likely to still be exercising a year later.

13.   **Nutrition.** Simple guidelines go a long way. A balanced diet low in fat and cholesterol will provide most of the nutrients you need. If not, take a multivitamin or supplements that are specific for your needs. Drink lots of water and eat as many high fiber foods as you can. Limit your intake of refined sugar. Eat iron and calcium rich foods. Don't skip meals. It causes your metabolism to burn calories less efficiently and actually can cause you to require fewer calories per day than if you were eating a more balanced diet in smaller, more frequent amounts. The portions you eat are worth keeping track of. Consult a dietitian to gain useful information, insight and direction.

14.   **Sleep.** Most of us need six to eight hours of sleep a night. Know what you need and plan your time so that you typically can get it. When we're really busy, trying to meet deadlines, or have young children, spending less time sleeping is the first way we try to create extra time. Once in while you can get along on less, but if it's a pattern, it can be injurious to your health. There's also the reality that as we age our sleep patterns become disrupted. A lot of literature is available with effective strategies to help you remedy simple sleep disturbances. Seek a professional if you need to.

15.   **Pay attention to your spiritual growth.** Are you a child or mature in terms of your spiritual development? Is your faith a first resort or a last resort when all else fails? What does it mean to be "spiritual"? Is being a part of a faith community important?

16.   **Challenge yourself intellectually and develop your intellectual curiosity.** Intentionally try to learn something new every day no matter how small or insignificant it may seem.

17. **Stay connected with healthy people.** Set time aside and plan for fun with people who can help you lighten up and enjoy some free time. Get out and do things you enjoy doing.

18. **Try a little "creative neglect"** with the "basement people" (we all have them) in your life especially when you are tired or handling too much. Don't become socially impaired by hanging out with people who influence you negatively when you don't have to be in their presence.

19. **Make sure you get enough "alone time."** How much time alone each of us needs varies, so find out what's right for you. Most caregivers spend a tremendous amount of time with others personally and professionally and relatively short periods of time alone. Check out the balance.

20. **Express your creativity** through music, painting, needle-work, sports, decorating, acting or whatever let's you share your-self from the inside, out.

21. If these common sense self help strategies aren't helping you create a healthier balance, **don't be afraid to talk with a friend or a professional counselor**. Telling your story, hearing yourself describe things to an attentive friend or professionally educated counselor can help you clarify your direction and put you back in balance again.

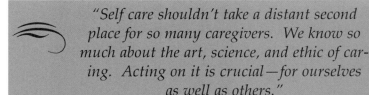

"Self care shouldn't take a distant second place for so many caregivers. We know so much about the art, science, and ethic of car-ing. Acting on it is crucial—for ourselves as well as others."
—*Diann Uustal*

◆ *Asking For What You Need And Want* ◆

Many of us have been conditioned for years not to ask clearly for what we need or want. Yet this is one of the most significant wellness concepts and strategies for taking care of oneself.

Maybe we don't ask because we're not sure what it is that we need or want. Or could it be that on some level we're afraid people won't respond to our requests? Think about various relationships you have or situations that arise and how it feels to ask the other person for something. "I need a hug , I'm feeling lonely." "I'm hungry, too, and right now, tired after being on my feet all day. If I could sit quietly for about 10 minutes , then we could start dinner together and talk." We all have these kinds of personal as well as professional requests and asking others to respond to us involves an element of risk taking.

This exercise is an opportunity for you to identify the things you need and want and to clarify the differences in your own mind between your needs and wants. You could even categorize them from a personal and professional perspective and pay attention to whether these needs and wants are emotional, social, spiritual, intellectual, or physical.

Remember, people can't read your mind! If you ask not, you have not!

Needs	Wants
1.	1.
2.	2.
3.	3.
4.	4.
5.	5.

What do you really **need more of** in your life?

•

•

•

What do you **want more of**?

•

•

•

What do you **need/want less of** in your life?

•

•

•

Are there differences between your "needs" and "wants"? What are the differences? (Ever tried to explain this to your kids in the Gap? Or when you really want something you know you can't afford?)

•

•

•

❋ **Fill in the following incomplete sentences. They'll help you think of other specific things you may need or want.**

1.   Someone in my personal life that I'd like more affirmation from is...

2.   Something I'd like to hear this person to say to me is...

3.   If I were to ask this person to validate a characteristic in me or notice certain qualities about me, I would ask for...

4.   One of the things I want most from my friends is...

5.   I'd like members of my family to...

6.   Someone I'd like more professional praise from is...

7.   I'd like to hear her/him say...

8.   Something I'd like more validation personally for is...

9.   I'm really working hard to...

10.   When my family/friends see me do this, I'd like them to...

11.   One thing I want to be remembered for is...

12.   Something I'd like my colleagues to notice about me is...

13.   A couple of things I'd really like more recognition for are...

14.   One thing I'd like to hear my son/daughter/best friend say to me is...

15.   In terms of my role at work, what I need most is...

✦ *Care Plans* ✦

We're all familiar with care plans, prescriptions, telegrams, FAXs and Email. It seems there are numerous ways for others to try to capture our attention. And they usually want it now. **With each style of communication, it seems as if the urgency of the message and the request for a response increases.**

The more urgent forms of communication help call attention to the immediate changes that are so necessary. They can help you with the balancing act that can be so tenuous some days. The strategies that call for planning might take longer to design and execute, but they will help you create a more balanced life.

So what is it you're after, a balancing act or a balanced life?

As a professional caregiver, you're familiar with care plans or care maps. Depending on your lifestyle or present circumstances, a balancing act may be just fine to bring you back to an even keel. For some people it would merely be a Band-Aid. What needs to be fostered is a balanced life. But first things first. Perhaps the following strategies will help.

We're good at writing care plans for other people's lives, but what about our own? What would a care plan for your life look like? What does your nursing diagnosis include and what are your professional recommendations? Don't forget to include physical, emotional, social, intellectual, and spiritual aspects. Start with steps that are manageable and meaningful to you.

Write at least the beginning of your care plan here:

Care Plan

Client's name:_____

Primary Care Provider: _____

Diagnosis:_____

Recommendations:_____

_____

_____

_____

A Prescription for Self Care

Prescriptions are usually written for us after a consultation with a healthcare provider and we fill them immediately in most situations. Maybe this serves as a good model for your reflection.

Write yourself a prescription. You've seen enough of them.

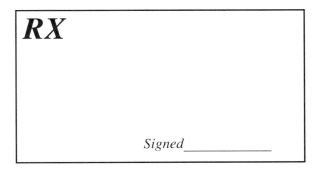

Will you fill the prescription?

Telegram

Maybe if a telegram were sent it to you would get your attention. Most of us can remember when they were an urgent form of communication. Go ahead, write yourself a telegram that starts off in the following way:

```
(    Your name    ), I URGE YOU TO:
```

FAX

FAX yourself a message. Snail mail, formal care plans, take time and telegrams are dated. Maybe you need to send a FAX containing some recommendations that you must pay attention to. Tell yourself specifically what you must do to stay healthy or get well. Give yourself some needed advice. Be your own consultant, after all you know yourself better than anyone else does. Write your FAX here:

Fax transmittal cover sheet

TO:
FROM:
DATE: # of pages:
Comment:

If fax is interrupted or illegible, please contact yourself again until you get the message.

Email

So what about Email? It has the advantage of being delivered as quickly as you can type the message and it can be extremely brief and direct. Write yourself an Email that will get your attention. What would your Email to yourself say? What would an Email from one of your friends who's concerned about your health or wellness look like? What's it going to take to get you to follow good advice?

To: Myself@whereIam.com
From: Me@whereIcouldbe.com
Subject: Stay healthy

You can complete any of these exercises or simply use them as a metaphor to help you take responsibility for your own health.

Here's some additional, simple wellness strategies and action steps you could take to help care for the caregiver:

- **Send yourself to your room once in a while for a "time out." This strategy may be familiar to you in terms of disciplining your children. What's wrong with a little self care discipline for yourself?**

- **Admit yourself to "intensive care" or the "recovery room."**

- **Go on a mini- retreat. Give yourself a little "re-creational" therapy. <u>No one can take care of you, except you.</u>**

- **Find a quiet place to rest and recover and care for yourself by doing something enjoyable or that refreshes you.**

You will be healthier from a holistic perspective and those around you will benefit too. You give your family advice all the time and give patients and their families the advantage of your professional recommendations.

Now take your own recommendations seriously.

 Rest isn't a luxury in your busy life.
It's a necessity.

♦ *Visualizing Wellness* ♦

There's an undeniable connection between your mind, body, and spirit. There's also a distinct relationship between your internal dialogue or self talk, the pictures you create in your mind, your perceptions of yourself, and your overall health and well being. **Practicing visualizing positive situations and affirming yourself enhances your wellness.**

Here are two visualization exercises that will help you practice. Read about them and then decide which one you'll try to visualize. Then sit or lie down in a place that's comfortable and quiet. Close your eyes. Slow yourself down and begin to focus on the visual strategy you have read about. Take some deep breaths, slow your breathing down, and consciously try to relax the muscles in your face, shoulders, arms, abdomen, and legs.

Visualization #1
Surround yourself with a color you enjoy.

What's your favorite color? See this color and imagine it as it spreads all around you. Identify the feelings you have when you see and experience this color. See if you can make the color brighter and then make it fade.

See if you can choose another color and do the same things. Choose as many colors as you like or go through a rainbow of colors. Don't rush through the visualization.

Open your eyes and take a few deep breaths or stretch. How do you feel? Are you more relaxed? In a few minutes, notice if you are able to focus more and if you are clearer in your thinking? Do you sense you have a little more energy available? You can use this exercise any time you want to help you relax. Teach it to others. Use it as a family strategy one evening.

Visualization #2
Imagine a place that's a harbor or shelter for you.

Close your eyes and imagine a place that's beautiful, peaceful and restful to you. It could be a place you've seen or never even been to. What do you see all around you? Look everywhere you can see in every direction with no interference. Just drink in the pleasure of being in this place.

Are you inside or outside? Are you sailing, on a beach, in a dance studio, gazing at a waterfall, in an elegant or simple room? Create the situation, the room or the view in any way you want.

What are you doing? Are you kicking back and enjoying this place? Are you alone? Who are the people there? Who else do you want to share this with? Take your time. You're in charge, this is your re-creation time.

Open your eyes slowly and come back to where you are. How did you feel physically, emotionally, and spiritually in that place? You can decide to go here any time you want. Use it anytime you need a mini-vacation.

In as little as 15 minutes you can visualize wellness. These mini-retreats are true refreshment breaks. It would be ideal to have a quiet room to go to for a break if you were at work. If you're at home, **send yourself to your room, or make a wellness appointment for yourself** where everyone knows and respects that this is a time out for you. If it's good enough for football, you can certainly use the concept!

It will take scheduling, perseverance, and respect (other people's and your own) in order set aside the time to accomplish this the first few times. Explain to your family that you need a short break in order to continue on. People who care for you will get used to it and perhaps even decide to follow your example.

The strategy rests on the fact that **in order to care for others, you have to know how and take the time to care for yourself and to recharge when you're tired. This is self respect not selfish.** Even Christ went into the desert to rest and pray first in order to prepare for the demands of the day. Who are your role models?

Here's another application for visualization: perhaps you can teach a person in pain to find additional relief by visualizing a comforting, safe place in order to get through a difficult procedure, or so that the medication is more effective or less is needed.

✦ *H a b i t s   T h a t   H u r t* ✦

Bad habits are hard to break and can compromise your wellness. Good habits don't come easy and sometimes you have to unlearn old patterns of behavior and thinking in order to become healthier. Look at the following sentences and ask yourself if they are never, seldom, often, or always typical of you. Use the numbers that indicate your response in front of each of the sentences.

1—never typical	**3—often**
2—seldom	**4—always**

___ 1. I feel guilty when I'm not working on or accomplishing something.

___ 2. I prefer to do most things myself rather than asking for help.

___ 3. I do two or three things at a time, such as talk on the phone, sort mail, eat.

___ 4. Things never get done fast enough for me.

___ 5. I spend a lot of time mentally planning and thinking about the future and as a result, tune out the here and now.

___ 6. I tend to put myself under pressure because of self imposed deadlines.

___ 7. It's hard for me to relax, even when I'm not working.

___ 8. I put more time, thought and energy into my work than I do into my relationships with family and friends.

___ 9. I get upset in situations where I can't be in control.

___10. I get very impatient when I have to wait for someone else or wait in line.

___11. Put your own idea(s) here.

Read the list again and check the habits that cause you more stress.

Prioritize at least two habits you want to remedy.

Choose one of them and decide what it is you could do or say when you find yourself in that situation the next time and sliding back into a habitual response.

For example, let's say you get irritated most of the time when you hear the phone ring. Sometimes you even answer too gruffly and sound impatient more often than not. You typically see the phone ringing as an interruption or you can choose to see it as someone who cares enough to want to spend some time with you (this does not include dinner time solicitation from an unknown individual selling a product you did not request!).

 "A bad habit never disappears miraculously. It's an un-do-it-yourself project."
—Abigail Van Buren,
Universal Press Syndicate

♦ *"Be-Friend" Yourself* ♦

When's the last time
you treated yourself like your best friend?

Think about your best friend. You try to do things for him/her that are special, that please her or make him feel good or cared for, right? You probably say things that are encouraging and uplifting. You listen with your heart to the things that are said and the feelings between the words that aren't even spoken.

Well here's a simple wellness strategy: *Treat Yourself Like You Treat Your Best Friend*. Try it for an hour or two, or the whole day, or even better, get in the habit of treating yourself well.

Be a friend to yourself. Be your own best friend.

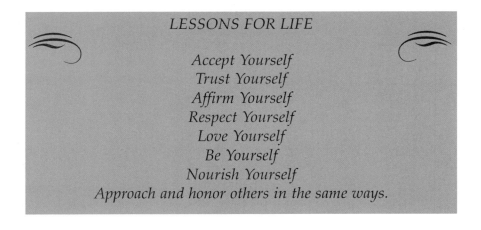

LESSONS FOR LIFE

Accept Yourself
Trust Yourself
Affirm Yourself
Respect Yourself
Love Yourself
Be Yourself
Nourish Yourself
Approach and honor others in the same ways.

♦ *Simple Strategies For Well-Being* ♦

Get some "Ventilatory Support"

Allow yourself to tell your story. Talking out your feelings to a caring person (your spouse, friend, family member) allows you a safety valve. Saying what you really think and feel is important and saying it to a person who won't betray the confidence is crucial. Face to face conversations are ideal, but phone calls may be helpful. Don't forget to be reciprocal in the relationship and be there when you're needed in return. Attentive listening to your partner is of equal value for both of you.

Be discriminating.

Sharing your feelings with too many people can also be stressful. You've seen this type of individual. Nothing goes unspoken about their trials and they wear themselves and others out. If this is you, recognize and adjust the pattern.

Who's your "chicken soup" person?

You need at least one, true-blue, trusted person you can count on when you need help. Who is a person who would be there for you no matter what time of the day or night? Would you do the same for him or her?

Know when to say when.

Commitment to a number of people who have issues can be exhausting and a burden too. Allowing too many people to turn to you as a primary resource when you're really stretched can be overwhelming. Be honest with them about your need to preserve your energy. It's not forever; it's a strategy for you to use when you're plate is too full.

Make your home a haven.

Your place should be a source of comfort and caring, yet for many of us it's a place where the tasks and demands seem endless. In addition, the TV and phone may invade your privacy or be sources of stress that prevent your family from talking with one another and sharing feelings about what's going on in their lives. Check out whether the things you "have to do" consume more time than the "recreation-al" time we need to set aside for ourselves and one another.

Create the life you want.

Do you know what you want in your life? What are you doing on a daily basis that moves you closer to creating this lifestyle? Do you need to take more time to think about what's of value to you? What would the conversation be like if your whole family were involved in discussing and planning this together?

Cultivate relationships that are healthy.

Intentionally spend time or call the people in your life who affirm, bring out the best, challenge, or respect you. Each person brings you special gifts (like a great sense of humor, encouragement, insight and friendship) and you have a chance to offer yours to them. They're your "balcony" people and we all need to be involved with healthy people.

Remember you're a human being, not a human doing.

Who are you? Do you define yourself primarily by your role? Wife, working mother, son, caregiver, single father, nurse, counselor, sister, uncle, social worker, godmother. The "Who am I?" question is an important one. For most of us, it's more complicated that it sounds. Forget your name or your role for a minute and just repeatedly ask yourself the question, "Who am I?" and jot down your responses.

Can you think about yourself and not associate yourself with any particular role? Is your sense of who you are so tied up with what you do, instead of who you are, that you've lost touch with yourself? You can be totally competent in your role and yet never take the time to answer the "Who am I?" question.

Readjust your focus. Bring others into focus.

One of the best ways to get past your own issues is to pay attention to other people in your life and get off your own story. Pay attention the next time you are listening to music or seeing a sunrise not only to the feelings you're aware of, but also the reactions of the person you are with. Work at discovering who you are based on your experiences with others.

◆ *"Spiritual Flat Tires"* ◆

Bernie Siegel, M.D. talks about "Spiritual Flat Tires" in his workshops. He says these spiritual flat tires are apparent setbacks. "Apparent setbacks" because it depends on how you define them or perceive them. An unexpected event can have a positive or a negative outcome based on how you choose to respond to it.

For example, my secretary and lifetime friend, BJ and I got in the car to go buy office supplies before the predicted snowfall accumulated any further. Most people were buying the usual: bread and milk. We were in a rush to meet some dead-lines and the weather had already forced a number of work days to be canceled which added to the urgency. The car wouldn't start. We both started spieling off a litany of complaints and happened to look up and see the tiniest snowflakes falling gen-tly on the windshield. They were absolutely perfectly formed. You could see how delicate and intricately detailed each was. Almost instantly we found ourselves marvelling at their beauty, trying to discover if there were any two alike, and even being grateful that it was snowing.

Thinking back to the event and the feelings of that day, I marvel at the timing and good fortune of being slowed down in the middle of a hectic day and at how good it felt to see such majestic art work, to know once again who was in charge, and to give praise for simple pleasures that offer respite.

The car surprisingly started up right after we had acknowledged, enjoyed, and celebrated.

I think the real spiritual flat tire would have been if we didn't respond to the beauty around us even though our plans were temporarily thwarted. Stop and smell the roses....or see the snowflakes....and give credit where credit is due...

So the next time an apparent setback occurs maybe you'll think of Siegel's "spiritual flat tires" and choose to respond in a way that decreases your distress rather than adds to it.

 "Such occurrences teach us to stop judging events as necessarily good or bad, right or wrong and, instead, just let life flow."
—*Bernie Siegel*

♦ *Are You As Happy As You Could Be?* ♦

When was the last time you really felt happy? Was it last year when you were on vacation? Your daughter or son's graduation? Moon shadows on the water? A friend's wedding? A relaxing meal? Does it take big things or little things to make you happy? This exercise is an opportunity to think about happiness in your past and present. Reflect on the following questions:

- *What do you mean by "happy"?*
- *What makes you happy?*
- *Is it elusive or pervasive in your life?*
- *If you could have more of it, describe what would it be like.*
- *Are you as happy as you could be?*
- *What needs to change?*
- *What are you doing to bring about these changes?*
- *Is happiness an attitude, or state of mind, or something external?*

We chase it, we erroneously equate it with money or success, and ignore the fact that people who have "things" aren't necessarily emotionally better off than the rest of us. H. Jackson Brown, Jr., the author of Life's Little Instruction Book has written: "People often confuse happiness with pleasure, and they're two different things. I know people who go out and try to buy happiness, but what they're really doing is buying pleasure, which doesn't last very long. You can go out and buy a new car and experience a great sense of pleasure, but after twenty minutes, twenty hours, or twenty days, the pleasure fades."

- *What's the difference for you between happiness and pleasure?*
- *Do you think you can buy happiness? Ever tried to do it? What was the result?*

Wayne Dyer the author of Real Magic: Creating Miracles In Everyday Life wrote: "Many people think happiness is something they can get from life. For instance, they're looking for happiness in their jobs or in their relationships. But happiness is not external; it's not what you get from life, it's what you bring to life. It isn't a thing, it's a belief. You can make the conscious choice to be happy at any time, and so, basically you are as happy as you make up your mind to be."

- *Do you think happiness is what you get from life or it's an attitude or belief as Dyer says?*

Wendy Kaminer, author of <u>I'm Dysfunctional, You're Dysfunctional</u> writes: "I think Americans feel entitled to be happy, and there's something very childish about that. It doesn't recognize how complicated life is and how much unhappiness and sorrow is a natural part of everyone's life; how much has to be managed, endured, and transcended. In fact, only through a certain amount of unhappiness can you learn what happiness really is."

- *Do you think Wendy is right? Why or why not?*

Webster's dictionary defines happy as lucky, fortunate. But don't you know plenty of people who are neither lucky nor fortunate and who are happy? They seem to have the capacity for en-joy-ment.

- *Do you have this capacity for enjoyment and happiness naturally?*
- *What do you think it would take to cultivate it in your life?*

Is feeling happier a matter of enjoying the people and things in your life more? Does it have to do with a general attitude you have toward life? Do you need to change anything?

- *Reflect on the moments of pleasure you experienced yesterday.*
- *How typical was the day for you?*

For children, happiness seems to have a magical quality and to be quite obvious to others. Studies of twins raised separately report that about 50 percent of our sense of well-being is inherited and the rest seems to be determined by our childhood and life experiences.

- *Recall some of the things that made you happiest as a child.*

Happiness to a teenager is often conditional and hinges primarily on excitement and new experiences. The peaks and valleys are still there, but the innocence of childhood happiness has changed.

- *What are some things, events, and people that brought you happiness as a teen?*

By the time we're adults, we've learned that the things that bring joy and happiness such as love, marriage, creating a family, and achieving career goals can also bring responsibility and loss.

- *What has added to your happiness as an adult?*
- *Have you found this happiness to be transitory?*
- *Is it more rare or frequent the older you get?*

What makes you really happy? Here are some responses from women and men in my workshops after we've worked through this strategy:

- *A good split between satisfying leisure time and challenging work.*
- *Having a weekend where I have time off.*
- *Reading for fun and not having a yellow underliner in my hand.*
- *Watching a sunset and listening to Kenny G.*
- *Swimming with the dolphins. That was inter-species happiness that was sublime. A lifetime memory!*
- *Holding our new granddaughter.*
- *Lots of messages at the end of the day when I come home on my answering machine.*

Happiness isn't just about what happens to us—it's about choices and how we think about what happens to us. It's the art of finding the positives to replace the negatives that can happen to any of us. It's the willingness to stop wishing for what we don't have, and enjoying what we do have. Our lives could be richer, more fulfilled and happier. The time to be happy is now.

 "We all live with the objective of being happy; our lives are all different and yet the same."
— *Anne Frank*

♦ *Life's Prizes* ♦

MOST OF US
MISS OUT
ON LIFE'S
BIG PRIZES.
THE PULITZER.
THE NOBEL.
OSCARS.
TONYS.
EMMYS.
BUT WE'RE
ALL ELIGIBLE
FOR LIFE'S
SMALL PLEASURES.
A PAT
ON THE BACK.
A KISS
BEHIND THE EAR.
A FOUR POUND BASS.
A FULL MOON.
AN EMPTY PARKING SPACE.
A CRACKLING FIRE.
A GREAT MEAL.
A GLORIOUS SUNSET.
HOT SOUP
COLD BEER.
DON'T FRET ABOUT
COPPING LIFE'S
GRAND AWARDS,
ENJOY ITS
TINY DELIGHTS.

Author unknown

- Can you think of any "life prizes" you feel you've missed?
- What are some of the things that bring you small pleasures?
- Is the last sentence of the poem good advice for you?

"Life's not about the day when you win the
prizes—it's about all the days in between."
—Susan Howatch, English Writer

◆ *An Attitude of Gratitude* ◆

Do you have an attitude of gratitude? Or are you typically aware of what's missing or wrong? Do you need to consciously "practice" being grateful and cultivating this attitude response to your experiences and life?

Spend some quiet time being thankful for the blessings you experience on a daily basis. It sounds silly, but start with the little things. For example, you don't have to remind your heart to keep a steady beat, your immune system to stay on top of things, or your big toe to keep you in balance. What a mess we'd be in if we had to coordinate all this. And you thought today was rough!

That's ridiculous, you say. Well, then think of other things that you're grateful for. If some of these involve a person, tell them in some way in the next few days how grateful you are that they are in your life.

 Complete this unfinished sentence *as many times as you can*:

I'm thankful for...

In the "Caring for the Caregiver" workshops I do, people have the opportunity to read what they're grateful for to the other members of the group. Let me share one person's response to this thankfulness strategy:

"I'm thankful for my past, my present and my future. I give thanks for everything that has happened in my life and the people who have crossed paths with me. All of these interactions have brought me to where I am today. I'm thankful for the here and now. I couldn't always experience it and I'm grateful I can do that now. This moment is one of contentment, relaxation, and peace and I realize how priceless this kind of joy is. I'm thankful for my future. It's a chance to grow more fully, to influence my family and friends in positive ways. I'm thankful that in God's eyes I'm perfect and that He loves me even though we both know I'm not."

 "I can complain because rosebushes have thorns...or rejoice because the thornbushes have roses...it's up to me."
—Anonymous

♦ *Change Is Good — Isn't It?* ♦

Change can be pleasurable or painful, welcomed or feared, an external or an internal force. Most of us consider change as a good thing unless it requires too much effort, someone else tells us it's good for us, or it's a situation we have little control over. In which case, we go kicking and screaming along with it, right?

Some changes seem to hold all these elements at once. Even when change is good it can still be stressful.

 What are some changes you've experienced in the past or been thinking about making in the future? Jot them in the appropriate spaces provided:

Pleasurable Changes

-
-
-

Painful Changes

-
-
-

Welcome Changes

-
-
-

Feared Changes

-
-
-

Self-Initiated

-
-
-

Other-Initiated

-
-
-

Loss of Control

-
-
-

Little Control

-
-
-

Think about one change you'd like or need to make. Write a few sentences describing the nature of the change and what's involved. Then answer the following questions about that change.

1. Will this change be pleasurable or painful or both?

2. What do you think will be different because of the changes you are making?

3. Are you ready for the changes?

4. Are you the one initiating this change or has someone else been telling you to change?

5. Do you feel you will have to deprive yourself because of this change or can you focus on what you will gain? For example, eliminating your favorite foods or the way you spend money might be two changes you need to make changes in. If you are concentrating on what you are depriving yourself of rather than on what you will gain, you'll have a more difficult time sticking to your plan. What do you need to forego and what do you expect to gain?

6. What are you unwilling to change?

7. Decide what you can cut out or what you can take on. (i.e. fat in your diet, increasing your exercise, etc.) Be as specific as you can.

8. What are the situations which tempt you or put you at risk the most for not sticking to what you want to change?

9. What qualities or characteristics do you need to exercise in order to be successful?

10. How can you keep up your motivation in order to be successful?

11. What are the values you hold that are the catalyst for the change you are making?

 "Everything we do, every decision and course of action we take, is based on our consciously and unconsciously chosen beliefs and values."
—*Diann Uustal*

♦ *In Order For Things To Stay The Same, Things Have Got To Change...* ♦

Intuitively, the message inherent in the title of this exercise rings true. We've all made resolutions, usually on a particular day of the year, or been determined to do something because of a specific occasion. Sometimes within days we re-discover that we're not living up to our best intentions or the goals we're striving for. Want to help yourself accomplish the change(s) you desire? Here is a strategy to get you thinking and give you some ideas to complete "A Contract With Myself" exercise in this book.

Why should you change? Good question. And it's a question only you can answer. Change in yourself doesn't come because someone else wants it for you.

❋ **Think about one change you need to make.** Now make a list of at least <u>10 reasons to make this change</u>:

1.   2.

3.   4.

5.   6.

7.   8.

9.   10.

Here are some success tips and strategies whenever you're serious about making a change:

- **Take small steps** toward the change you want to make. For example, reduce the number of fat grams in your next meal, limit your cigarettes to one fewer a day each day for a week, walk on the treadmill for five minutes every other day the first week.

- **Choose a date** when the specific plan will begin. Stick with the changes you want and don't make exceptions. For example, you can still eat out or attend a dinner meeting and stick to your diet.

- **Announce it to everyone** so that they'll give you support or challenge you to stick to your plans, which will help you reach your goals.

- **Make a plan** for what you'll do when you don't have the "won't power" or "will power" to stick with your goal. For example, when you want that desert, or don't feel like exercising. When the old pattern creeps in, put your plan into action.

- **Call someone** on your support team **if you feel you're wavering or about to "relapse."** Call them to get validation for the successes you are having, too.

- When you've achieved your goal, **celebrate your success** in the way you said you would and have a contract burning party! Be sure to celebrate and "own" your success.

- **Establish a new contract** if you need or want to.

- Instead of a "New Year's approach" to change, **start immediately with a few changes you really desire.** Set your self up for success by being as specific, practical, and consistent as you can. If you fall short of your goal, as soon as possible, start again. **Be sure to celebrate your commitment to change and your success!**

✦ *Assets And Liabilities* ✦

The business world operates on the principle of maximizing the assets and minimizing the liabilities. On a psychological level, you can utilize this principle as a means of increasing self concept and self esteem and intentionally focusing on personal strengths rather than weakness. Your "assets" are your abilities, strengths and talents. "Liabilities" are the things you need or want to change, not things you think are negative about yourself. In the space below make a list of your assets and liabilities:

My Assets (abilities, strengths, talents)	My Liabilities (things I need to change)
•	•
•	•
•	•
•	•
•	•
•	•
•	•
•	•

Now that you've completed these two lists, answer the following questions:

1. Did you find it was easier to identify your assets or your liabilities?

2. Why do you think this is so?

3.   Go back and read your list and rank in order the liabilities you identified in terms of the degree to which they typically can interfere with either your assets or your achievements. Number one is the most interfering and so on.

4.   Choose one of the liabilities you identified. What can you realistically do to limit the influence of this liability? Be as specific as you can.

5.   Make a list of your personal and professional accomplishments, achievements, and successes. Go ahead, don't be hesitant.

Accomplishments, achievements and successes	Assets that helped
•	•
•	•
•	•
•	•
•	•
•	•

6.   Next to each accomplishment, identify the asset(s) that were instrumental in helping you achieve.

7.   Which liabilities do you need to change because they are keeping you from achieving as much as you are capable of?

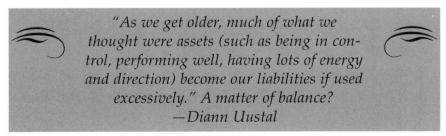

"As we get older, much of what we thought were assets (such as being in control, performing well, having lots of energy and direction) become our liabilities if used excessively." A matter of balance?
—Diann Uustal

♦ *Invest In Yourself* ♦

Most of us are very familiar with basic financial strategies and principles. For example, when you deposit and leave money in your bank account, it accrues interest over time. When you need some money, you can make a withdrawal from your account. But what if you haven't made a deposit in a long time and you've made repeated withdrawals? There's less capital available when you need it, the interest earned is less, and if the withdrawals continue with no deposits, your account will be overdrawn.

This metaphor doesn't stretch the imagination too far when you use it to evaluate how well you're taking care of yourself. If you don't take the time to "take care," and don't invest in yourself in some consistent, self caring ways, then you'll begin to find that the constant withdrawals will deplete your account. Sure you can live on the interest, for a while, as long as the demands don't cost too much, aren't too frequent, or for too long.

So if you want to stay healthy or get healthier and you want to care for others well, then take the time to invest in yourself. Don't forget to think of yourself from a whole person perspective and that you have physical, emotional, intellectual, social and spiritual sides of you to care for and invest in. Don't get caught in a recession or depression. Invest wisely and for the long term. The dividends will pay off!!

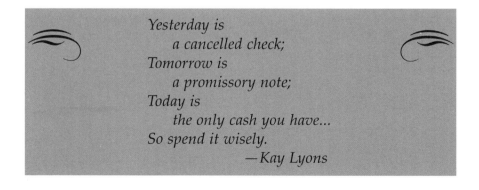

Yesterday is
*   a cancelled check;*
Tomorrow is
*   a promissory note;*
Today is
*   the only cash you have...*
So spend it wisely.
*   —Kay Lyons*

◆ *Care Coupons* ◆

One time our younger daughter, Katie, presented me with a "care coupon" which tickled me. It read:

> *This coupon is*
> *good for dusting.*
> *One time.*
> *Without complaining!*

She signed her name and it came with an expiration date!! I've never thrown that coupon out and still hold it up for people to see in my workshops.

Here are some examples of Care Coupons we've used for fun.

> *You deserve a treat today!*
>
> *At your favorite entertainment, feast, or gift place, too!*
> *Just name it and I'm treating you!*
>
> *Just present yourself and this coupon.*

You may want to place some limits on this next one!

> *Need a favor?*
> *No coupon is necessary for you.*
> *But just in case it's hard to ask,*
> *Bring this along and we'll see what we can do!*

> *If It's Not Unethical,*
> *Illegal ,*
> *or Fattening*
> *You've Got It!*
> *Just Flash This Coupon.*

Need a massage?
Your feet are tired, your shoulders ache?
Say no more.
You'll enjoy!
Just present this coupon and start relaxing.

(You can return the good deed as soon as I'm through.)

Need someone to talk to?
I've got two ears and one mouth.
And your story goes no where else.
You know you don't even need this coupon—
It's just a visual reminder...
And an offer to listen.

"Your care for others is a measure of your own greatness."
—Luke 6:48
Thanks for your caring.
What goes around comes around—I owe you one!

I read this today: "I am only one; but I am still one. I cannot do
everything, but I still can do something. I will not refuse to do the
something I can do." (Helen Keller)
Thinking of you and hoping to help...

 Make up and share some of your own Care Coupons
and enjoy.

◆ *Don't Become A Victim* ◆

Psychologists have discovered that many caregivers, women, and minorities experience oppression in their personal relationships or in the systems in which they work more frequently than the general population. Among the many understandable reactions and feelings, these individuals often see themselves as victims.

In his book, "The Three Boxes of Life—and How to Get Out of Them," Richard Bolles, a minister and career counselor writes that buying into "...the victim mentality is the biggest cause of people failing to find satisfying work." He defines the victim mentality, as an outlook or attitude in which a person says, "My life is essentially controlled by powerful forces (or a vast powerful force) outside of me and beyond my control." Therefore, they believe they are governed by:

- history, upbringing, genes, or heritage

- social class, education (or lack of it) or I.Q. (or lack of it)

- parents, teachers, or a relative

- husband, wife, partner

- boss, supervisor, manager, or co-workers

- the economy, times they live in, social structure, or government

- politicians, large corporations, or the rich

- some particular enemy who is out to get them and has a lot of power

Read the list carefully and then check off the ones you experience as oppressive. Bolles has found that usually at least four of these areas are selected if an individual is struggling with experiencing satisfying work or the victim mentality. Use these categories to reflect on areas that you may want to examine and change. Devise a plan that will help you deal more directly with particular situations you find limiting or people who exert more influence and control than necessary. This kind of plan and change is never easy, but it will help add to your wellness and self care.

◆ *Making Decisions:*
Who's In Charge? ◆

Each of us is constantly making decisions and some of these are more important than others. They may be as simple as what to wear or eat, how much allowance is appropriate for your child, or as complex as whether to return to graduate school, or not to resuscitate a patient who doesn't want to be resuscitated even though her physician refuses to write a No CPR order.

All decisions are made on the basis of beliefs and values; however, most of us have difficulty identifying what we really believe as opposed to what others advise us to think or do.

 Think about a recent personal or professional decision that was difficult for you to make. Or think of a difficult decision you know you'll have to make in the future. Briefly describe it here:

1. What values helped (or will help) you make your decision? Write them here.

2. What values were in conflict in your difficult decision? List them here.

3. Imagine that you are the chairperson of an advisory committee and that you are meeting to decide the best way to handle your decision. Who will you appoint to advise you? List their names.

4. Why would you select these people to be on your advisory committee? What qualities, skills, insights, or values do they have? Identify as many as you can for each person.

5. What would each person "advise" you to do concerning this dilemma?

6. What "should" messages do you hear from them?

7. Are you the "Chairperson" of your committee or is there another person in charge? What do you need to do if someone else is in charge of your decisions?

8. Is there someone you'd like to add to your advisory committee?

9. Is there someone you'd like to remove?

10. Draw a picture of the table at which you and your advisory group are sitting. What shape does it have? Where are you sitting in relation to the others? Do either of these variables have any effect on your decisions?

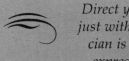 *Direct your life with meaningful choices, not just with efficiency or speed. The finest musician is the one who plays with passion and expression, not the one who finishes first.*

◆ *Goal Setting* ◆

When you identify and set goals for yourself, they should meet the 3 M's of goal setting if you want to ensure the possibility of achieving them. Your goals should be measurable, manageable, and meaningful.

❋   There are many areas of your life that you may want to examine more closely as you establish your goals. Rank order these areas from 1 to 8 in order of importance to you.

____attitudes toward and about yourself

____family life

____job satisfaction

____personal relationships

____physical fitness

____spiritual growth

____stress management

____ _____(your own alternative)

•   Write one *goal* you'd like to achieve:

•   What are some *barriers*, blocks to change, ways you might sabotage yourself from reaching your goal?

•   What are some *actions* you could take to minimize these barriers?

- Who are some *people* who could help you reach your goals?

- What are some other *resources* that could help you reach your goals?

- What do you *expect, want* from these support people?

- What *payoffs/positive results* do you expect when you reach this goal?

- What *negative results* might occur if you reach this goal?

- What do you have to do to *decrease the negative outcomes*?

- Do the *positive outcomes outweigh the negative outcomes*?

- Do you *still want to work* toward achieving this goal?

- If you want to achieve your goal, *list the steps* you need to take to reach this goal

- List the *qualities you need* to reach this goal.

♦ *"Dear Career . . . "* ♦

Psychologists have encouraged their clients to write letters to either individuals or inanimate objects to help the client clarify feelings and examine thoughts and values that are often unexpressed. It's a letter that doesn't have to be mailed, but it serves as a springboard for growth and a mirror for personal reflection. Writing to the problem as if it were able to understand is a surprisingly effective strategy and it's a healthy way to begin to deal with certain issues and feelings that can emerge.

 So why don't you try this strategy? Write a letter to your job, career, or profession. Don't edit your thinking. Go ahead, tell your career what you think about:
- what you'd really like to be able to do
- what you're unhappy with and want to change
- what the stressors are
- the goals you have
- conflicts in values you experience.

Let your thoughts and feelings find expression and if it helps include:

1. things you like about your job, career, or profession

2. values you're able to express

3. some things you want to accomplish in your position

4. some professional goals you have

5. stressors in your role or profession

6. conflicts in values in your job

7. things you'd like to learn or do

8. strategies you use to cope in your position

9. changes you'd like to make to improve the quality of your professional experience

10. risks you'll have to take

11. what brings you the most satisfaction

You could adapt this strategy and write a letter to almost any person or situation and then ask yourself some clarifying questions. It might be an effective tool for sorting out your feelings and allowing them to be expressed in a safe way. You may want to work on the letter over time and then send it on.

If you are using this exercise in a group setting, ask for volunteers to read their "Dear Career" letters to the group. When I ask for volunteers in my workshops, it's always a powerful exercise that creates tremendous camaraderie. It can serve as a catalyst for discussions about how the work environment can be changed, what the caregiver's values are, and how the system can interfere with what many of us really want to accomplish.

Remind the group of confidentiality issues and support those colleagues who are taking the risk of sharing these letters. Validate your colleagues who have shared their thoughts.

Ask some clarifying questions that relate to job role and satisfaction that the group can respond to such as:

1. What could you do to increase your satisfaction with your career?

2. What could the manager on the unit, or in your agency do to:
   > —enhance job satisfaction
   > —wellness in the workplace
   > —nurse-nurse collegiality and interdisciplinary collaborative practice and collegiality

3. What can you do to decrease the stress of your role?

4. What does your ideal role/career look like?

5. Is nursing a job, a career, or a profession to you?

◆ *A Contract With Myself* ◆

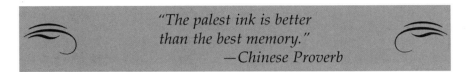

*"The palest ink is better
than the best memory."*
—Chinese Proverb

Identifying something you want to change, putting it in writing like AT&T says, and having someone witness your intent are often useful incentives toward accomplishing your goal. Make a contract with yourself and post your written intent where it can serve as a reminder.

It could be something physical, emotional, financial, social, spiritual, intellectual, or a character trait or habit that you want to change. So make a deal with yourself and contract for change and ask someone who will validate your efforts to encourage you throughout the process. Remember to reward yourself for your progress, no matter how small and celebrate your achievements.

I,_____do promise to commit myself to achieving the following goals and activities. This agreement is with myself, and is being witnessed by a supportive friend so that I can achieve success. This contract will be in effect from:

_____to_____

One thing I especially want to change is...

My plans and activities for accomplishing this goal are...

Indications that I am meeting my goal are...

Ways in which I might sabotage myself or prevent myself from reaching this goal are:

I will do my best to eliminate these by:

Ways in which I can reduce or eliminate my patterns of self sabotage are:

The person who will help me keep my contract with myself is_____.

I plan to reach my goal by_____. A copy of this contract is shared with those who will encourage me to keep my contract with myself.

The rewards I'll relish when I reach my goals are:

What I'll do to celebrate my success when I reach this goal is:

Signed:_____
          (Your name)

Signed:_____
          (Trusted Witness)

Date:_____

"What you have is a plan.
The rest is life..."
—*Rev. Tom Thompson*

♦ *Making Your Contract With Yourself Work!* ♦

 "Don't make promises you can't keep!"

Didn't your Mom and Dad raise you on this value? How many times do we promise ourselves to do or change something? Then somehow we don't keep that promise to ourselves even when we know it's important.

You can make your contract with yourself work more effectively by being even more specific about your expectations and goals. Below are some things you may want to change and some revealing questions that will help you think about how your can keep your promises. Let's say you want to:

1. Lead a more active lifestyle.

A fine goal, but be specific about how you will work more activity into your already crowded day.

> In order to increase my activity by _____ minutes a day, I will:

Here are some possibilities for you to consider:

- substitute a "coffee break" with a "movement break" at least twice a week
- walk the stairs or walk outside
- get off the bus one stop early or park further away from where you're going
- don't use the remote control on the TV for the weekend

- temporarily or permanently get rid of some of the labor saving devices you've accumulated.

2.   Make exercise fun and non-routine.

Cross train and get your cardiovascular exercise by doing lots of different things because you know how boring the same old thing can be. For example, plan to go dancing instead of doing a half hour on the stair stepper again. Complete the following statements:

- I can't even stand the thought of:

- so instead I'll get my aerobic activity by:

One of my friends borrowed his son's in line skates and now delights in skating, weather permitting, in the mall parking lots before the crowds arrive.

3.   Eat a whole lot healthier.

You wouldn't put the wrong fuel in your car, so why would you put the wrong fuel in your body? You can't trade it in for a new one. Again, be specific about how you're going to do make this change.

- To eat healthier, I am going to:

- I will eat more:

- and less:

- Three things I won't give up are:

  1.

  2.

  3.
- but I'll limit the amount of times I indulge in them without guilt to _____ a week.

4.   **"Lighten-up" and set realistic goals.**

Change is difficult. We often set our goals too high or give ourselves too little time to accomplish them. Then the unachieved expectations understandably make us feel as if we've failed or we're inadequate. For example, let's say you were going to exercise 30 minutes a day, four days a week. Why not say you'll "do something physical" at least four days a week? By slightly revising the goal, you might have more success sticking with it and achieving what you want.

- Write your goal here:

- What you can do to achieve it is:

- Some realistic strategies for increasing your chances for success are:

5.   Reduce or eliminate the patterns that compromise your health.

What are the things you're doing that put more stress on your already taxed body and mind? Do you use too much alcohol to relax, smoke to unwind and control your appetite, too much caffeine to deliver a burst of energy? Do you work too much? Look at your patterns that could be diminishing your vitality.
- What are the patterns that compromise your health?

  -

  -

  -

  -

- What are the "benefits" you get from these patterns? What are the burdens to your overall wellness and health from these patterns?

  Benefits   **Burdens**

  -                                -

  -                                -

  -                                -

  -                                -

- Choose a pattern you'd be willing to try to change.

I can change or reduce_____

_____

to _____ times a week. I can stop doing _____

_____and substitute _____

_____instead.

6. Create a better balance, not just a "balancing act."

Take the quiet time to feed your soul and nourish your spirit. Find out when the best time to take this quiet time is. Protect it as sacrosanct. Do pleasurable things even if it's only for a few minutes a day at first. Talk to a friend, pamper yourself by doing something relaxing or alone for 15 minutes. Schedule something that's fun and that you look forward in your calendar. Now set up the rest of the demands of your day around this "appointment".

- Some things I can do for fifteen minutes that will fit into even my day are:

- One thing I can do by the end of this week to pamper myself is:

7. Reach out and touch.

Find a way to give something back each day. There is a tremendous benefit that you can experience when you are altruistic and take a little time and energy to concentrate on others who also need care.

If you truly do not have the energy for this, don't feel guilty. You are the one who needs intensive care. But when you do have a little more to give, you'll find it's meaningful and re-energizing to give of yourself. You'll probably receive more than you share. Maybe you could teach adults in your community to read, call someone and leave them a validating voice mail message, help serve at a food kitchen, collect shoes and coats for the homeless shelter, or "adopt" an elder at a nursing care facility as a friend or a new grandparent.

- I'd be willing to reach out and give back by:

◆ *Just For Today I Will...* ◆

Here are some of the comments that have been shared by participants in my workshops after they have interacted together using a number of different strategies. "Just for today I will..." is a strategy that can be the first step you take before you complete a contract with yourself and hold yourself to some of the changes for a longer period of time. See how many of these participant responses you would find helpful in making some of the changes you want to make.

"I will do the best I can in a situation and then discipline myself not to worry about it."

"I create additional stress for myself lots of times. One way that doesn't work is that I try to control others and my subjective response is all I can really control. That's where the real control is and I need to do that better."

"I will do one thing at a time. Well maybe just two instead of my usual overload."

"I will think and live positively, committing myself to being the best I can be."

"I will try to learn from even from bad experiences."

"I will express my feelings honestly to other people. This has never been easy for me. I'm always worried about what others might think."

"I will treat others with the respect I want for myself."

"If I or my partner are dissatisfied with a particular aspect of our relationship, I will take steps to improve it rather than settle for a less qualitative relationship."

"Death is a normal, inevitable part of life. I know and accept this. I will embrace and celebrate life wherever I can."

"I will pay attention to my own needs and try more deliberately to

respond to them and not feel guilty about it."

"I will work at not feeling closed in and will focus on the options I have available and can create."

"By paying attention to my needs physically, emotionally, and spiritually, I will choose to be well and happy."

"I will live in the here and now. I will stay in the room."

 Now that you've read your colleague's responses, what would you say you'd try to do "just for today?"

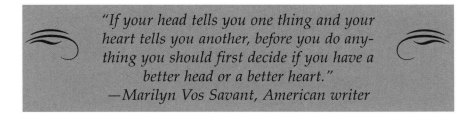

"If your head tells you one thing and your heart tells you another, before you do anything you should first decide if you have a better head or a better heart."
—Marilyn Vos Savant, American writer

◆ *When I Am Old* ◆

My wonderful college roommate and present-day friend, Karla, creates beautiful cross stitch art work. One year for my birthday, in graduated shades of purple, she cross stitched this poem which has been a favorite of mine for years.

When I am an old woman I shall wear purple
With a red hat which doesn't go, and doesn't suit me.
And I shall spend my pension on brandy and summer gloves
And satin sandals, and say we've no money for butter.
I shall sit down on the pavement when I'm tired
And gobble up samples in shops and press alarm bells
And run my stick along the public railings
And make up for the sobriety of my youth.
I shall go out in my slippers in the rain
And pick the flowers in other people's gardens
And learn to spit.

You can wear terrible shirts and grow more fat
And eat three pounds of sausages at a go
Or only bread and pickles for a week
And hoard pens and pencils and beermats and things in boxes.

But no we must have clothes that keep us dry
And pay our rent and not swear in the street
And set a good example for the children.
We must have friends to dinner and read the papers.

But maybe I ought to practice a little now?
So people who know me are not too shocked and surprised
When suddenly I am old, and start to wear purple.

—by Jenny Joseph

- What do you need to "practice" a little more?

- No matter what your age, do you have to wait until you're older to do some of the things you want to do?

- What changes have you already been making that add to the quality of your life?

◆ *Taking Care of Yourself* ◆

Love yourself. Accept yourself. Don't be so hard on yourself. Now do this for others. Love your neighbor as yourself becomes easier when you give this gift to yourself.

Think about what you most want out of your life. Ask the people you love what they want.

Genuinely affirm and validate people in your family, your friends and colleagues each time you see them for their characteristics as well as for the things they're doing things well.

The past is over, concentrate on what you've learned and what you can do differently now because of what you've learned. You don't have to repeat the past.

Treat yourself to personal or alone time to enhance your wellness.

Change the way you typically do things to help stay out of a rut. Take a new way home. Surprise yourself and do things upside down and backwards once in a while.

Keep your promises to yourself. Do what you say you're going to do "when you get some free time."

Experience and pay attention to all your feelings. Allow and encourage others to do the same.

Celebrate life once in a while by doing something you really love doing.

Ask yourself, "Am I being authentic right now? Am I living in ways that are congruent with my values? Am I staying in touch with who I am and want to become from a holistic perspective?" Then take action based on your responses.

Consciously try to live a life of simplicity and balance rather than one of complexity and chaos. Pay attention to what helps or hinders you in striving for this peace.

Take some quiet time each day to reflect on the things and people in your life that really count and add to the quality of your life. Count these as blessings and be sure to communicate your gratitude.

Think about the wake up calls you've had in your life! What did you learn? Are you remembering the lessons you learned?

Be a collector of memories not just things.

Frolic regularly and learn to play or be impulsive for fun. Be silly and ridiculous once in a while.

Write a validating letter to yourself. Write one to someone you love. Write one to someone who needs it. How about writing one to someone you're in conflict with? (Now that's a hard one!)

Be ahead of your time. Be visionary.

Invent ways to surprise or show you love or care for someone.

Feel rich without any money.

Be your self.

Drink in all the sunsets, sunrises, and moon shadows you can.

Pay attention to your intuition and insight.

Invite yourself out to play.

Create friendship rituals you share with special folks.

Create a family, friendship, or happiness journal and record what's happened to make you happy. Read and recall the good times regularly together. Create more of them.

Invite some friends over and tell life stories.

Take your shoes off and walk in the grass or on the beach.

♦ *"T i m e - O u t !"* ♦

"Time out!" It's a familiar demand that even athletes who are in peak condition use during a game to stop the clock, regroup, and make a new game plan. Parents even use "time outs" as a disciplinary strategy to help their children gain some control, slow down, and reflect on a situation. Caregivers can certainly profit from using this concept as a wellness strategy.

When's the last time you declared a "time-out" so that you could collect your wits or muster additional energy? Imagine that you could actually do this during a pressing day at work.

Instead of going for a coffee break, which may have questionable benefits for your health, or to a cramped locker room, wouldn't it be nice to really relax for the few minutes you have? Imagine that a room has been designed so you can go there to relax and unwind. It's a place where you can be comfortable, rest, and take some time for yourself. It's quiet, carpeted, and there are comfortable places to sit and put your feet up. The best part is that you can listen to your favorite music on the Walkmans that are amply available in the room. Maybe you and your colleagues could call this "intensive care" or the "comfort zone."

Why is this type of setting, where caregivers can truly relax, even if it's only for a brief time, just in our imaginations? Wouldn't a place like this make sense for nurses and other caregivers to retreat so that they can re-energize? This is not a place for team meetings, conferences, lunch, or conversations with your colleagues. It is a serene environment where you can rest briefly and re-create so that you can continue to care effectively.

I've introduced this idea in my workshops and to hospitals I consult with throughout the country. In one area, a public advertising campaign associated with Nurse's Week was launched in the newspaper. It proposed ways for the community to thank nurses for their excellence in caring. The response by the public was overwhelmingly positive! Numerous Walkmans, the carpeting and floor pillows were donated by individuals and local businesses, and even the labor involved in creating the room was donated. A tape library was started with the money generated by the "Thank a Nurse Today" fund described in the newspaper. The gratitude for nurses and nursing by members of the community was evident. "Ask and you will receive!" was the principle that was the foundation for this simple strategy to reduce caregivers' compassion fatigue! Try it and see if something like this will work in your community.

Of course you could also use this strategy on a personal level too. Declare a time out for yourself periodically. Send yourself to your room! Sometimes you will only have a few minutes, other times longer. Create a space and some time so that you can refresh and get back in balance.

◆ *If I Had My Life*
To Live Over ◆

I'd dare to make more mistakes next time.
I'd relax, I would limber up.
I would be sillier than I have been this trip.
I would take fewer things seriously.
I would take more chances.
I would climb more mountains and swim more rivers.
I would eat more ice cream and less beans.
I would perhaps have more actual troubles,
but I'd have fewer imaginary ones.

You see, I'm one of those people who lives
sensibly and sanely hour after hour, day after day.
Oh, I've had my moments, and if I had it to do over again,
I'd have more of them. In fact, I'd try to have nothing else.
Just moments, one after another,
instead of living so many years ahead of each day.
I've been one of those persons who never goes anywhere
without a thermometer, a hot water bottle, a raincoat and a parachute.
If I had to do it again, I would travel lighter than I have.

If I had my life to live over,
I would start barefoot earlier in the spring
and stay that way later in the fall.
I would go to more dances.
I would ride more merry-go-rounds.
I would pick more daisies.

—Nadine Stair

- If you had your life to live over, what would you do differently?
- What would you do more of? Less of?
- What things would you take less seriously?
- What chances would you be willing to take?
- What troubles would you create fewer of?
- What moments would you try to experience more of?
- What's missing in your life?
- What makes you happiest?

 Don't worry about what you could do if you lived your life over. Get busy with what's left.

♦ *Take Time* ♦

Take time to work.
It is the price of success.

Take time to meditate.
It is the source of power.

Take time to play.
It is the secret
of perpetual youth.

Take time to read
It is the way to knowledge.

Take time to be friendly.
It is the road to happiness.

Take time to laugh.
It is the music of the soul.

And take time
to love
and be loved.

—Adapted from an old Irish prayer

"Time is like a series of liquid transparen-
cies. You don't look back along time,
but through it, like water.
—Margaret Atwood, Canadian writer.

♦ *In Closing* ♦

I hope you've enjoyed reading this book and interacting with the material and trust the exercises have been practical and useful in helping you assess and create a balance between caring for yourself and caring for others that's right for you--not just a balancing act, but a balanced life.

I believe self care enhances the quality of your caring for the people in your personal life and the value of your therapeutic relationships with your patients and clients. In order to continue caring empathetically for others, you must negotiate, weigh, and balance caring for yourself and caring for others.

This book shared numerous ideas and strategies for enhancing your wellness from a holistic perspective, increasing your self esteem, and promoting healthy caring in your personal and professional relationships. My hope is that you will take the ideas that make sense to you and translate them into action.

Keep it in mind that:

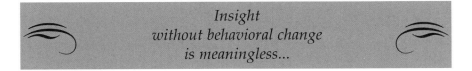

*Insight
without behavioral change
is meaningless...*

Take care! Your caring counts!

♦ *A b o u t t h e A u t h o r* ♦

Diann received her B.S. in nursing from the University of Rhode Island, and her M.S. in nursing from the University of Massachusetts. She earned her Doctorate at the University of Massachusetts in Education, majoring in the area of ethics and values in health care. In 1994, Dr. Uustal completed a year's post doctoral fellowship in clinical-bioethics as a Visiting Fellow at the Kennedy Institute of Ethics at Georgetown University.

Diann is the founder and president of an educational consulting firm, Educational Resources in HealthCare, Inc. and is a nationally and internationally recognized educator, author, and consultant. Dr. Uustal is a facilitator of workshops and seminars in clinical ethics, professional caregiver issues, and values education which are presented to hospitals, colleges of nursing, and various professional nursing and medical organizations. Diann was inducted into Sigma Theta Tau, the National Honor Society in Nursing in 1973 and has served as President of two different chapters and been a member of the National Nominating Committee.

Diann has received numerous awards and recognition outside the profession of nursing including: Who's Who of Women Executives in 1989; Outstanding Young Women in America in 1992; and International Who's Who of Professional & Business Women in 1994; and Who's Who of American Women for 1997-1998. In addition, she was named to Who's Who in American Nursing in 1993; one of Ten Most Outstanding Graduates of the University of Rhode Island, College of Nursing in 1995; and the Outstanding Alumni in Nursing at the University of Rhode Island in 1997.

As a clinical-ethicist, Dr. Uustal is experienced in consulting with hospital ethics committees, conferring in problematical clinical-ethical cases, reviewing and writing policies, and helping establish new ethics committees. Diann has authored numerous articles in health care values and ethics, professional issues in nursing, and caring for the caregiver.

Diann has written four books; the two most recent are entitled Caring for Yourself ~ Caring for Others: The Ultimate Balance and Clinical Ethics and Values: Issues and Insights in a Changing Health Care Environment. She has also co-edited two books entitled Cutting Edge Bioethics: A Christian Exploration of Technologies and Trends and Teacher Burnout. In addition, Diann was a major consultant for the award winning Concept Media film series on Ethics, Values and Health Care and wrote the script for the film entitled "Values Clarification."

Dr. Uustal's workshops and contributions in the areas of the ethic of care, ethical issues in health care, and caring for the caregiver are widely recognized in the nursing and medical professions. She is a highly sought after educator, author and keynote speaker, known for her dynamic and thought provoking presentation style.

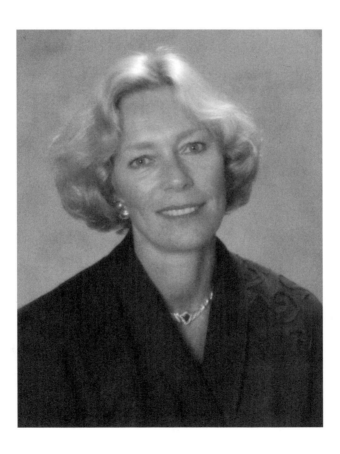

◆ *References* ◆

Angelou, M. (1969) <u>I know why the caged bird sings</u>. NY: Bantam.

Ardell, D. (1977) <u>14 days to a wellness lifestyle</u>. Mill Valley, CA: Whatever Publishing.

Babbitt, D. (1993) <u>Downscaling: Simplify and Enrich Your Lifestyle</u>. Chicago: Moody Press.

Bach, R. (1977) <u>Illusions</u>. NY: Dell Publishing Co.

Beattie, M. (1987) <u>Codependent no more</u>. San Francisco, CA: Harper & Row.

Belenky, M.F., Clinchy, B., Goldberger, N.R. & Tarule, J.M. (1986) <u>Women's ways of knowing</u>. NY: Basic Books.

Benner, P & Wrubel, J. (1989) <u>The Primacy of Caring</u>. Menlo Park, CA: Addison-Wesley Publishing Co.

Bern, E. (1964) <u>Games people play</u>. NY: Grove Press.

Biehl, C. (1990) <u>I can't do everything</u>. Sisters, OR: Questar Publishers, Inc.

Biro, B. D. (1997) <u>The Joyful Spirit</u>. NY: Pygmalion Press.

Blanchard, K. & Johnson, S. (1981) <u>The one minute manager</u>. NY: Berkley Books.

Bleier, R. (1984) <u>Science & gender</u>. NY: Pergamon Press.

Branden, N. (1995) <u>The Six Pillars of Self-Esteem</u>. NY: Bantam.

Brothers, J. (1978) <u>How to get what you want out of life</u>. NY: Simon & Schuster.

Burns, M. (1982) <u>Run with your dreams</u>. Greenville, MI: Empey Enterprises.

Buscaglia, L. (1972) <u>Love</u>. NY: Fawcett Crest.

Canfield, J. & Wells, H.C. (1976) <u>100 ways to enhance self concept in the classroom</u>. N.J.: Prentice Hall.

Canfield, J., Hansen, M., Aubery, P. & Mitchell, N. (1996) <u>Chicken soup for the surviving soul</u>. Deerfield Beach, FL: Health Communications, Inc.

Carlson, R & Shield, B. (1989) <u>Healers on healing</u>. Los Angeles, CA: Jeremy P. Tarcher.

Carlson, R. (1997) <u>Don't Sweat the Small Stuff... and It's All Small Stuff : Simple Ways to Keep the Little Things from Taking over Your Life</u>. NY: Hyperion.

Chinn, P. (1991) <u>Anthology on Caring</u>. NY: National League for Nursing Press.

Cousins, N (1987) <u>The pathology of power</u>. New York: WW Norton Co.

Cousins, N. (1979) <u>Anatomy of an illness</u>. NY: Bantam Books.

Cousins, N. (1983) <u>The healing heart</u>. NY: Avon Books.

Covey, S. (1989) <u>The 7 habits of highly effective people</u>. NY: Fireside.

Covey, S. (1994) <u>First things first</u>. NY: Fireside.

de Saint, Exupery, A. (1943) The little prince. NY: Harvest/HBJ Books.
Dubrin, A. (1997) Getting It Done : The Transforming Power of Self-Discipline. Princeton, NJ: Peterson's Guides.
Dyer, W. (1976) Your erroneous zones. NY: Avon.
Eisenberg, R. & Kelly, K. (1997) The Overwhelmed Person's Guide to Time Management. NY: Plume.
Elgin, D. (1993) Voluntary Simplicity : Toward a Way of Life That Is Outwardly Simple, Inwardly Rich. NY: Quill.
Elkins, D. (1976) Glad to be me. N.J.: Prentice-Hall, Inc.
Ferguson, M (1980) The aquarian conspiracy. Boston: GK Hall.
Fulghum, R. (1988) All I really need to know I learned in kindergarten. NY:Villard Bks.
Fulghum, R. (1988) It was on fire when I lay down on it. NY: Ivy Books.
Gaut, D & Leininger, M. (Ed.) (1991) Caring: the compassionate healer. NY: National League for Nursing Press.
Goldberg, M (1983) The intuitive edge. Los Angeles: JP Tarcher.
Harris, T. (1968) I'm OK, you're OK. NY: Continuum Pub. Corp.
Hay, L. L. (1997) Empowering women : Every woman's guide to successful living. Carlsbad, CA: Hay House.
Held, V. (1993) Feminist Morality. Chicago, IL: University of Chicago Press.
Herman, S. (1978) Becoming assertive: a guide for nurses. NY: Van Nostrand.
Howe, L. (1979) Taking charge of your life. Niles, IL: Argus.
James M. & Jongeward, D. (1971) Born to win. Reading, MA.: Addison-Wesley.
Jampolsky, G. (1970) Love is letting go of fear. NY: Bantam.
Jolley, W. (1997) It only takes a minute to change your life! NY: St Martins Mass Market Paper.
Jongeward, D. & Scott, D. (1976) Women as winners. Reading, MA.: Addison -Wesley.
Jourard, S. (1964) The transparent self. NY: Van Nostrand.
Kaufman, B. N. (1994) Happiness is a choice. NY: Fawcett Books.
Keating, K. (1983) The hug therapy book. Minneapolis, MN.: CompCare Pub.
Kim, S. H. (1996) 1,001 ways to motivate yourself and others. Wethersfield, CT: Turtle Press.
Kushner, H. (1981) When bad things happen to good people. NY: Avon Books.
Lair, J. (1975) I ain't well-but I sure am better. Greenwich, CT.: Fawcett Crest.
Lakoff, G & Johnson M (1980) Metaphors we live by. Chicago: University Press.
Lakoff, G (1987) Women, fire & dangerous things. Chicago: University of Chicago Press.

Leininger, M. (Ed,) (1984) <u>Care: The essence of nursing and health</u>. Detroit, MI: Wayne State U. Press.

Leininger, M. (Ed.) (1988) <u>Care: Discovery and uses in clinical & community nursing</u>. Detroit, MI: Wayne State U. Press.

Leininger, M. (Ed.) (1988) <u>Caring: An essential human need</u>. Detroit, MI: Wayne State U. Press.

Linbergh, A. (1965) <u>Gift from the sea</u>. NY: Vantage Books.

Little, B. (1978) <u>This will drive you sane</u>. MN: Camp Car Books.

Maslow, A. (1961) <u>Toward a psychology of being</u>. N.J.: Van Nostrand.

Mayeroff, M (1971) <u>On caring</u>. NY: Perennial Library.

McWilliams, P. (1995) <u>You can't afford the luxury of a negativethought</u>. NY: Prelude Press.

Meissner, J. (1986) <u>Nurses: Are we eating our young?</u> Nursing 86 51-53.

Miller, JB (1976) <u>Toward a new psychology of women</u>. Boston: Beacon Press.

Montagu, A. (1971) <u>Touching: The human significance of the skin</u>. NY: Harper & Row.

Moustakes, C. (1977) <u>Turning points</u>. N.J.: Prentice Hall.

Mueller, M. K. (1997) <u>Taking Care of Me : The Habits of Happiness</u>. NY: Insight Inc..

Munsch, R. (1986) <u>Love you forever</u>. Willowdale, Ontario: Firefly Books.

Naisbitt J & Aburdene P (1990) <u>Megatrends 2000: Ten new directions for the 1990's</u>. New York: William Morrow.

Naisbitt, J. (1982) <u>Megatrends</u>. NY: Warner Communications.

Newman, M. & Berkowitz, B. (1971) <u>How to be your own best friend</u>. NY: Ballantine Books.

Norwood, R. (1989) <u>Women Who Love Too Much: When You Keep Wishing and Hoping He'll Change</u>. Parkridge, IL: Parkside Medical Services.

Paulus, T. (1972) <u>Hope for the flowers</u>. NY: Paulist Press.

Peale, N. (1974) <u>You can if you think you can</u>. Greenwich, CT: Fawcett Crest.

Peale, N. (1982) <u>Positive Imaging</u>. Pawling, NY: Foundation for Christian Living.

Pearsall, P. (1996) <u>The Pleasure Prescription : To Love, to Work, to Play Life in the Balance</u>. Hunter House.

Pearsall, P. (1997) <u>Write Your Own Pleasure Prescription : 60 Ways to Create Balance and Joy in Your Life</u>. Alameda, CA: Hunter House.

Peisner, P. (1992) <u>Finding Time : Breathing Space for Women Who Do Too Much</u>. Naperville, IL: Sourcebooks Trade.

Peters, T. & Waterman, R. (1982) <u>In search of excellence</u>. NY: Harper & Row.

Pines, A. & Aronson, E. (1988) <u>Career burnout, causes and cures</u>. NY:

Free Press.

Powell, J. (1969) <u>Why am I afraid to love</u>. Niles, Ill: Argus.

Powell, J. (1969) <u>Why am I afraid to tell you who I am?</u> Niles, IL: Argus.

Powell, J. (1970) <u>The secret of staying in love</u>. Niles, Ill: Argus.

Prather, H. (1971) <u>Notes to myself</u>. NY: Bantam Books.

Rechtschaffen, S. (1997) <u>Time Shifting : Creating More Time for Your Life</u>. New York: Doubleday.

Rogers, C & Stevens, B. (1967) <u>Person to person</u>. NY: Real People Press.

Rogers, C. (1961) <u>On becoming a person</u>. Boston: Houghton Mifflin Co.

Rogers, C. (1977) <u>On personal power</u>. NY: Dell Publishing.

Rubin, T. (1989) <u>The Angry Book</u>. Parkridge, IL: Parkside Medical Services.

Salzberg, S. (1997) <u>Lovingkindness : The Revolutionary Art of Happiness</u>. Boston: Shambhala Publications.

Satir, V. (1972) <u>Peoplemaking</u>. Palo Alto, CA: Science & Behavior Books.

Schuller, R (1985) <u>The be (happy) attitudes</u>. Waco, TX: Word Book Publisher.

Schuller, R. (1983) <u>Tough times never last, but tough people do!</u> NY: Bantam Books.

Selzer, S. M. (1996) <u>Life's little relaxation book</u>. NY: Crown Pub.

Sheehy S. (1981) <u>Pathfinders</u>. NY Bantam Books.

Sheehy, G. (1976) <u>Passages</u>. NY: Bantam Books.

Siccone, F & Canfield, F. <u>101 ways to develop student self-esteem and responsibility</u>. Deerfield Beach, FL.: The Self Esteem Store.

Siegel, H (1986) <u>Love, Medicine & Miracles</u>. NY: Harper & Row.

Siegel, H. (1989) <u>Peace, Love & Healing</u>. NY: Harper & Row.

Simon, S, & Kirchenbaum, H. <u>Values Clarification</u>. Niles, IL: Argus.

Simon, S. (1973) <u>Meeting yourself halfway</u>. Niles, IL: Argus.

Simon, S. (1974) <u>Caring feeling, touching</u>. Niles, IL: Argus.

Simon, S. (1976) <u>I am lovable and capable</u>. Niles, IL; Argus.

Simon, S. (1977) <u>Vultures</u>. Niles, IL: Argus.

Simon, S. (1978) <u>Negative criticism</u>. Niles, IL: Argus.

Simon, S. (1988) <u>Getting unstuck</u>. NY: Warner Books, Inc.

Simon,S. & Simon, S. (1990) <u>Forgiveness</u>. NY: Warner Co.

Smith M. (1975) <u>When I say no, I feel guilty</u>. NY: Dial Press.

Sontag, S (1990) <u>Illness as metaphor and AIDS and its metaphors</u>. New York: Doubleday (originial work published in 1978 & 1988).

Toffler, A. (1977) <u>Future shock</u>. NY: Bantam Books.

Toffler, A. (1980) <u>The third wave</u>. NY: Bantam Books.

Uustal, D. (1978) <u>Values and ethics: considerations in nursing practice</u>. Amherst, Mass: Educational Resources in Nursing Press.

Uustal, D. (1985) <u>Values and ethics in nursing: from theory to practice</u>. E. Greenwich, RI: Educational Resources in Nursing & Wholistic Health.

Uustal, D. (1987) <u>Values: the cornerstone of Nursing's Moral Art.</u> <u>Ethics At the Bedside</u>. Philadelphia, PA: J. B. Lippincott.

Uustal, D. (1989) Caring for the Caregiver. <u>Nursing Network</u>. Berkshire Medical Center, Vol I, No.1, May, 1989, p4-5.

Uustal, D. (1991) Caring for yourself as you care for others. <u>Healthcare Trends and Transition</u>. Vol 2, No 5, April.

Uustal, D. (1991) RX: holistic caring for the caregiver. In B. Dossey, Guzzetta, C, Kenner, D (Ed) <u>Critical Care Nursing: Body-Mind-Spirit</u>. Scott, Foresman/Little Brown.

Uustal, D. (1992) The ultimate balance: caring for yourself~ caring for others. <u>Orthopaedic Nursing</u>. Vol 11, No 3 , May/June.

Uustal, D. <u>Clinical ethics and values: issues and insights in a changing healthcare environment</u>. (1993) East Greenwich, RI: Educational Resources in HealthCare.

Viscott, D. (1989) <u>The Language of Feelings</u>. Parkridge, IL: Parkside Medical Services.

Watson, J. (1985) <u>Nursing: the philosophy & science of caring</u>. Boulder, CO: Colorado Associated University Press.

Watson, J. (1988) <u>Nursing: human science and human care</u>. Denver, CO: University of Colorado Health Sciences Center.

Wegscheider-Cruse, S. (1987) <u>Learning to Love Yourself</u>. Deerfield Beach, FL: Health Communications, Inc.

Weisinger, H. & Lobsenz, N. (1981) <u>Nobody's perfect (how to give criticism and get results)</u>. NY: Warner Books.

Wholey, D. (1997) <u>The miracle of change : The path to self discovery and spiritual growth</u>. NY: Pocket Books.

Wilson, P. (1997) <u>The little book of calm</u>. NY: Plume.

Wirths, C. (1994) <u>Choosing is confusing : How to make good choices, not bad guesses</u>. Palo Alto, CA: Consulting Psychologists Press.

Zukav, G. (1989) <u>The seat of the soul</u>. New York: Simon & Schuster.

Order your copies of Dr. Uustal's audiotapes and books now!

BOOKS
$24.95 per copy plus $5.00 for postage and handling:

_____ copies of **Clinical Ethics and Values: Issues and Insights in a Changing Healthcare Environment**

_____ copies of **Cutting Edge Bioethics: A Christian Exploration of Technologies and Trends**

_____ copies of **Caring for Yourself—Caring for Others: The Ultimate Balance**

AUDIOTAPES
Numerous educational tapes are available in the areas of health care ethics, caring for the caregiver, wellness, leadership/management, and collegiality. The list below includes the title only. For a complete description of the audiotapes and a brochure, please call: 423-451-0011.

1 Care-based Ethics: Clinical Ethical Decision Making in Contemporary Health Care
2 End of Life Decisions: The Ethics of Clinical Ethical Decision Making
3 The Ethical Challenges Raised in Managed Care
4 Pain, Pain, Go Away! The Ethics of Pain Management & Palliative Care
5 Assisted Dying: Compassion or Conundrum?
6 When is Enough, Enough? The Ethics of the Futility Debate
7 Nutritional Support/Hydration: Ordinary or Extra-Ordinary Treatment?
8 Quality of Life – Sanctity of Dying: Humane Perspectives on Difficult Choices
9 Caring for the Caregiver: A Wellness Retreat for Nurses
10 Attitudes Are Contagious: Are Yours Worth Catching?
11 Chaos or Clarity: Values & Ethics That Should Shape Healthcare Reform
12 Value-Based Leadership: Character Counts!
13 Must They Suffer to Death? Improving End of Life Care
14 Nursing: A Job, A Career, or A Ministry?
15 Caring for Yourself – Caring for Others: Life on Fast Forward!
16 A Dignified Future: Ethical Issues in Caring for the Elderly
17 The Medicalization of the Living Room: Ethical Issues in Home Health Care
18 Whose Choice is it Anyway? The Ethics, Process, & Politics of Healthcare Decision Making
19 From Etiquette to Ethics: Nursing's Traditions, Transformation & Leadership
20 The Ethic & Spirit of Care

1 tape @ $10.^{00} + $2.^{00} P & H   3 tapes @ $26.^{00} + $5.^{00} P & H
12 tapes @ $81.^{00} + $9.^{00} P & H   All 20 tapes $125.^{00} + $12.^{00} P & H

Ship by return mail to:

Name _____

Address _____

City, State, Zip _____

Payment in full must accompany all orders. Please make checks payable and send to:

Educational Resources in HealthCare, Inc.
(From September through May each year)
2168 S. Shore Acres Rd.
Soddy Daisy, TN 37379
Phone: 423-451-0011
Fax: 423-451-0005

Educational Resources in HealthCare, Inc.
(From June to August each year)
PO Box 574
Jamestown, RI 02835-0574
Telephone: 401-423-1711
Fax: 401-423-1211

Please contact Dr. Diann Uustal if you would like her to design and present a multidisciplinary ethics workshop customized to meet your group's needs, or a specifically designed caring for the caregiver/wellness workshop, or to consult with your ethics committee.